INTERMITTENT FASTING FOR WOMEN OVER 50

The Easy, Natural Way To Lose Weight, Detox Your Body, Have More Energy And Slow Down Aging

TABLE OF CONTENTS

INTRODUCTION

What is intermittent fasting?

Intermittent fasting involves alternating periods of feast and famine in which you may eat as much as you like during the feasting but drink only water during the fast. The aim is to achieve the benefits of calorie reduction and for some, use it as vehicle to lose weight.

Intermittent fasting can be done over a number of days, in alternating 24 hour periods or daily. The first option reuires you abstain from some or all meals on one or more days of the week. Daily fasting utilizes 24 hour periods of eating and fasting that begin an end at the same time each day, for example fast from Monday 6pm until Tuesday 6pm, eat as much as you like from Tuesday 6pm to Wednesday 6pm and repeat the process. During daily intermittent fasting there is a short period for eating, usually 4-6 hours within the 24 hour day during which you can eat as much as you like.

Some of the things that put people off are the fear that they will be extremely hungry and not stick to the plan or do not know how to fit it into their schedule. This is actually quite simple if you plan in advance you get eat your evening meal at pretty much the same time everyday but at an hour either side depending if on an intermittent fasting phase or an eating phase. Again with a little planning you can also accommodate socializing and eating out.

The main factor preventing many people from trying is the fear of being hungry. Although this does take a little will power and a slight degree of discomfort to begin with it is actually quite easy!

There have been a number of studies over the past few years that look into the health benefits of fasting or intermittent fasting. Here is a review of some of the benefits and drawbacks of intermittent fasting.

- **Helps reduce weight**

There are a lot of diet plans out there and most of them talk about reducing your calorific intake and replace meals. The problem is that when the diet is over and you have reached your goal it is easy to go back to old habits and put the weight back on. Intermittent fasting is more of a lifestyle change and a slow burn diet. One of the most popular intermittent fasting diets is the 5:2 plan. Here you eat normally for 5 days and reduce your calorie intake for the other 2. There are many ways you can do this, you can eat nothing for 24 hours or reduce calorie intake to just drink fluids or very light meals. Obviously your 2 days shouldn't be back to back, spread them throughout the week.

- **Blood Pressure, Insulin and Cholesterol**

Numerous studies have shown that intermittent fasting will help reduce Cholesterol and Insulin which helps break down body fat and boost your energy. Furthermore, intermittent fasting can reduce the body's resistance to insulin which significantly lowers the risk of type 2 diabetes. Intermittent fasting has shown to relieve stress and high blood pressure that are both key risks for heart disease. When we fast a few days a week the body goes through a process that renews old cells and provides protection against various diseases.

- **Effect on the Brain**

Intermittent fasting can help the brain recover □uickly and stay healthy. Reduction in blood sugar and reduced inflammation increase your brain hormones which will keep you alert and focused. As well as helping the brain it prevents diseases that affect the brain such as

Alzheimer's. Fasting can help delay the onset of this degenerative disease.

Potential Risks of Fasting

The most common risk from intermittent fasting is dehydration. If you are consuming less than your body is taking on less water, it is very important you don't forget to drink on the days you do not eat. Water is essential and black coffee is often used if you get bored with plain water. With no food going in the stomach you are at risk from heartburn from stomach acid and long-term ulcers that can occur if stomach acid builds up against the stomach walls. The mental side of fasting also has to be considered. If you fast 2 days a week don't over indulge on the other 5, keep to normal meals or it could lead someone to psychological disorders such as bulimia. You also need to be sure you are eating the right nutrients and minerals. Continue to eat fruit and vegetables. If you don't eat for 2 days, make sure they other 5 you are eating enough fruit and vegetables and not just binge or convenience foods.

Intermittent Fasting For Beginners

Intermittent fasting for beginners has two rules to follow:

1) ***Fasting has to be pleasurable and NOT stressful.***
2) ***Fasting has to be simple and NOT rigid.***

From an experienced faster's standpoint, I have a few suggestions for intermittent fasting beginners. There are two major reasons for people who want to do intermittent fasting (IF) - weight loss or health or both. In any case, it's good to observe these two formulas:

More rules = more complicated = ***low chance of success***

Less rules = less complicated = ***high chance of success***

In terms of health, a 24 hour period off of eating is very healthful, it helps you reduce calories without sacrificing what you like to eat on your non-fasting days, and maybe even more importantly it stimulates your body to produce more growth hormone. Yes that's right growth hormone, the same one you hear about the celebrities taking to 'stay young'. Growth hormone has many anti aging benefits, and one of the most interesting being fat burning!

How to do Intermittent Fasting?

In an ideal situation, 2 sessions of 24-hour fasts in a week will be good enough to produce significant health and weight loss benefits. However, for beginners, you are not recommended to jump start with a 24-hour fast, unless you are absolutely sure that you can do it. There is no standard rule of doing IF. Simply try it and make it works for you. Let simplicity and flexibility be your fasting motto. Don't make it stressful for yourself.

As a beginner to practice intermittent fasting, I would say 'clear your mind from any other weight loss methods and focus on IF'. This is your first step towards IF success. Think how many times you've been told that breakfast is the most important meal in a day or you need to eat 6 to 10 small meals a day in order to lose weight. I'm not saying these rules are wrong. If these rules work for you, stay with them. But if you are setting your feet onto the route of intermittent fasting, better put these concepts aside at least for the period you are trying out IF. Having your IF mindset ready? Then begin with 'skip meal' and see how your body responds. I would say this is the simplest and easiest way to begin your intermittent fasting journey.

Pick a day to try 'skip breakfast'. Have fresh juice, water or tea instead. No coffee please. If that works out fine, try 'skip lunch' and move on progressively. A 24-hour fast can be done by anybody with an appropriate fasting mindset. One useful tip is not to think of food. Avoid social talk at the pantry over lunch hour. Go out for a walk or do some simple exercises.

<u>You can also explore these **IF** options:</u>

- Condensed eating window, e.g. eat ONLY between 11am and 5pm;
- Skip meal on an unplanned basis, as far as it is natural and not interfere your daily work;
- Early and late, i.e. skip lunch;
- One meal a day, ideally dinner only when you are relaxed and really have time to enjoy food.

To repeat, fasting has to be pleasurable and not stressful. Don't press hard on yourself. Be flexible. This is very important. Don't upset your boss when you are called upon a business lunch by telling him that you are fasting. Do it as you see fit and your schedule permits.

Is Fasting Safe?

With regards to losing weight, one method has become much more widely used in recent years and that method is fasting. Fasting isn't a new idea, in fact quite the opposite, it is probably one of the oldest methods of weight control there is, although that is a completely different story altogether.

The □uestion of whether or not fasting is safe is one that has been posed many times, more often than not by the medical and nutritional experts of the day although both fields are now starting to be a lot more open-minded about this often controversial method of losing weight. So is fasting safe?

In general, fasting involves the self-deprivation of food, li□uids or both. Then again, fasting may come in different kinds like water only, fruit or vegetable juice fasting, intermittent, etc. But, in many cases, individuals will totally abstain from food intake. Unfortunately, when talking about achieving goals of rapid weight loss, the answer to the □uestion. Is fasting safe, this is not as cut and dry as many would hope that the answer is both yes and no!

As for everything else in life, most things are fine in moderation and fasting is no different. If you fast for too long then the effects can be negative causing illnesses and conditions ranging from anorexia to liver failure, but fasting for comparatively short periods of time but on a regular basis can provide many benefits including colonic health and clearer skin as well as weight loss.

Although it is a 100% true that the many types of fasting will help people to lose weight pretty □uickly, it can also be true that a lot of that weight would be fluids and not fat, well at least initially anyway and only if you were in a total fast, that's when you consume no water and no food, not recommended by the way!

Benefits Of Intermittent Fasting

Insulin resistance, the most prominent feature of type 2 diabetes, has long been known to improve with caloric restriction. After a period of fasting, insulin sensitivity rises, and insulin levels fall. These result in improved fasting and postprandial glucose levels.

Also, as insulin induces adipose tissue growth, there is less propensity to weight gain and potentially even weight loss. Insulin resistance is associated with an increased inflammatory state including elevated C-reactive protein, decreased adiponectin, lower low-density lipoprotein (LDL) particle size, and other metabolic factors that all contribute to or are associated with atherosclerosis and development of coronary artery disease.

Furthermore, insulin is known to be both atherogenic as well as increase the risk of fluid retention and congestive heart failure. Thus, reducing insulin levels through intermittent fasting would have the potential for reducing major adverse cardiovascular events. Such a reduction in insulin may be achievable. It was reported on three patients who were able to discontinue insulin treatment 5–18 days after beginning intermittent fasting, during which they ate dinner but skipped breakfast and lunch on either alternate days or 3 days per week.

Further investigation of this hypothesis in larger populations is needed, but this finding is a tantalizing and potentially paradigmshifting result if it can be safely and reliably repeated in large populations.

Intermittent fasting and calorie restriction have been shown to improve various metabolic and inflammatory pathways. Included are increased heat shock protein, promoting cellular autophagy, reducing advanced glycation end products, increased adiponectin, and decreased inflammation cytokines. Each of these effects result in decreased vascular dysfunction and would, therefore, be expected to improve cardiovascular risk and/or mortality.

The Fat-Busting Benefits of Intermittent Fasting Include:

1. **Increased Growth Hormone.**

This was one of the main benefits that really interested me. Many people think little of their hormones unless a doctor has specifically told them that they have a hormone disorder. But our hormones are incredibly important. One of these hormones, most commonly known as the human growth hormone, is vital for our weight. This hormone is produced within our pituitary gland and is responsible for maintaining bone density, brain health, the health of our tissues, increasing muscle mass, and promoting the regeneration and growth of cells.

When you are undergoing a fast, this hormone will naturally increase to high levels within your body. Studies have found that it can raise up to five times its normal level While your hormones need to remain balanced, it is both safe and ideal to increase the human growth hormone. This is because this hormone, sometimes shortened to HGH, often reduces as we age, predisposing us to increased body fat, decreased muscle, and more delicate and thinner skin. Yet, when we increase this hormone studies have found that we can experience greater fat loss, increased muscle strength, stronger bones, and strengthened cardiovascular health.

2. Converts White Fat into Brown Fat

One amazing aspect of intermittent fasting is that it not only helps you lose fat, but it converts your unhealthy white fat into a much healthier (and important) brown fat Many people are unaware that there are multiple types of fats within our bodies. But, while white fat is known to contribute to disease and aging, brown fat protects our organs and helps our bodies to burn off the white fat. This, of course, leads to weight loss, but also to increased health.

3. Reduced Muscle Loss

I used to think that if I reduced my overall calories then I'd just lose bodyfat. Nope. That's wrong. Yes, I lost some bodyfat, but I lost hard earned muscle mass too. Yikes! People often get excited about weight loss when they begin a crash or fad diet. But what most don't realize is that this weight loss is mostly water weight which will only return and all-important muscle loss. Not only are our muscles important for our strength and energy levels, but our heart is even a muscle Thankfully, a study published in 2011 found that while both intermittent fasting and calorie restriction lead to comparable fat loss, intermittent fasting lead to much less muscle loss than the calorie restriction did.

4. Boosts Energy Levels

The human body is full of cells. Some of these cells are known as mitochondrial cells, which can produce energy from multiple sources. These sources of fuel include protein, fat, carbohydrates, and ketones. While some cells may only be able to utilize one or two of these fuels as an energy source, mitochondrial cells are able to utilize all these fuels.

This is especially wonderful news for people who are on a low-carb diet because the brain and a few other cells re□uire glucose from carbohydrates in order to be fueled. However, when you are fasting or in a state of ketosis, your body will naturally produce an increased number of mitochondrial cells, helping you to use other fuel sources for energy within the brain. While the mitochondrial cells may not replace all of your cells that re□uire glucose for fuel, you can still stay satisfied and healthy when fasting or on a ketogenic diet. This is because of the process of gluconeogenesis.

This process converts amino acids from the proteins we eat into the small amount of glucose these nonmitochondrial cells require. Between the increase in mitochondrial cells and a healthy amount of fat and protein between fasting periods, you will find your body is well-fueled despite going longer periods without eating.

5. Lower Chronic Inflammation

Inflammation is a daily part of life and aids in keeping our body healthy. The immune system uses inflammation in order to treat injuries and prevent infections. Yet, some people develop high levels of inflammation which may become chronic. These cases of chronic inflammation are becoming more widespread with the modern diet, lack of sleep, too much work, and the stress of modern living. While inflammation may be a beneficial and necessary component of our immune system when used in moderation, when it is increased in this way it becomes dangerous.

Not only does increased levels of inflammation increase sleeping difficulties, pain, and many other symptoms, it can also increase the risk of disease. Studies have found chronic inflammation levels can lead to cancer, rheumatoid arthritis, heart disease, and more. Thankfully, intermittent fasting has been shown to help resolve these problems. By following a fasting schedule for one month, participants within a study were able to lower their inflammation levels greatly. Another study found the same results when people practice daily twelve-hour fast for a month.

6. Cell Repair

Intermittent fasting has been shown to increase autophagy. This is a critical role within our bodies which help replace our old and decaying cells with younger and healthy cells. The point of this is to keep our bodies functioning in a homeostatic state. If autophagy isn't active enough, then we can develop diseases. The process is so powerful that researchers are searching for a way to increase autophagy with drugs, to help treat people with chronic and terminal diseases. By intermittent fasting you can increase this vital process naturally, helping to increase your lifespan and lower your risk of developing diseases. Studies have even found that it can help your stem cells activate into a state of self-regeneration.

7. Oxidative Stress Reduction

We commonly develop oxidative stress through our environment, food, lack of sleep, and even though the process of transmuting food into fuel and energy. When we develop oxidative stress and free radicals it travels throughout our bodies and damages healthy cells. This in turns leads to disease and an increased rate of aging. However, we can combat the process. Studies have found that by practicing intermittent fasting, we are able to reduce oxidative stress and increase the antioxidants that fight against it.

CHAPTER ONE

METABOLISM AND HOW IT WORKS

Metabolism is the complex biochemical process by which the food you eat is converted into the energy your body needs to function. That, in a nut shell, is what metabolism is. Most people look at their metabolism in a more simplistic sense and see it as the thing that influences how their body will gain or lose weight. There are many things that affect our metabolism, from the composition of each individual body to the food we eat and how active we are.

Every living thing gets the energy it needs from the food, or nutrients, it eats. The human body is no different. Without food we run out of fuel and our metabolic engine, the body, stops working. There is more to metabolism then just converting nutrients into energy. It also aids in the digestive process and the absorption of nutrients into the cells as well as breaking down and removing harmful substances, such as drugs, poisons, and alcohol from the body.

There are specific proteins in the body that control the chemical reactions of metabolism and each chemical reaction is coordinated with other body functions. There are several hormones produced by the endocrine system that control the rate of the metabolic process. Thyroxine, which is a hormone produced and released by the thyroid, plays a key role in determining how fast or slow the chemical reactions of metabolism occur in the body.

There are two basic components of metabolism. The first is Anabolism, or constructive metabolism, which is the building and storing function of the metabolic process. It supports the growth of new cells, the maintenance of body tissues, and the storage of energy (fat storage) for future use. The second component is Catabolism, or destructive metabolism, which is the process that produces the energy required for all activity in the cells.

During this biochemical process, calories -- from carbohydrates, fats and proteins -- are combined with oxygen to release the energy your body needs to function. The number of calories your body burns each day is called your total energy expenditure. Even when your body is at rest, it requires energy for the basics, such as fuel for organs, breathing, circulating blood, adjusting hormone levels, plus growing and repairing cells. Typically, a person's basal metabolic rate is the largest portion of energy use, representing two-thirds to three-□uarters of the calories used each day. For the most part, your body's energy requirement to process food stays relatively steady and isn't easily changed. Weight gain is more likely due to an energy imbalance -- consuming more calories than your body burns.

Skipping meals or reducing caloric intake by a large amount is not a good idea either, because the body will actually slow its metabolism to conserve energy. Creating a demand to burn more calories is the best way to increase metabolism. People who exercise on a regular basis naturally can eat more food without gaining weight because they use more calories. When the body is not supplemented with additional calories, as when the person eats a normal healthy diet, this tends to increase metabolism with resultant weight loss.

Metabolism is a necessary process, without which living organisms would die and it is important to not only know what is metabolism, but to also take care of your body so that your metabolism is able to remain consistent.

Nutrition, Metabolism And Energy

Nutrition is the key to metabolism. The pathways of metabolism rely upon nutrients that they breakdown in order to produce energy. This energy in turn is required by the body to synthesize new proteins, nucleic acids (DNA, RNA) etc.

Nutrients in relation to metabolism encompass bodily requirement for various substances, individual functions in body, amount needed, level below which poor health results etc.

Essential nutrients supply energy (calories) and supply the necessary chemicals which the body itself cannot synthesize. Food provides a variety of substances that are essential for the building, upkeep, and repair of body tissues, and for the efficient functioning of the body.

The diet needs essential nutrients like carbon, hydrogen, oxygen, nitrogen, phosphorus, sulfur, and around 20 other inorganic elements. The major elements are supplied in carbohydrates, lipids, and protein. In addition, vitamins, minerals and water are necessary.

Carbohydrates In Metabolism

Foods supply carbohydrates in three forms: starch, sugar, and cellulose (fiber). Starches and sugars form major and essential sources of energy for humans. Fibers contribute to bulk in diet.

Body tissues depend on glucose for all activities. Carbohydrates and sugars yield glucose by digestion or metabolism.

The overall reaction for the combustion of glucose is written as:

$$C6H12O6 + 6\ O2 \longrightarrow 6\ CO2 + 6\ H2O + energy$$

Most people consume around half of their diet as carbohydrates. This comes from rice, wheat, bread, potatoes, pasta, macaroni etc.

Proteins In Metabolism

Proteins are the main tissue builders in the body. They are part of every cell in the body. Proteins help in cell structure, functions, haemoglobin formation to carry oxygen, enzymes to carry out vital reactions and a myriad of other functions in the body. Proteins are also vital in supplying nitrogen for DNA and RNA genetic material and energy production.

Proteins are necessary for nutrition because they contain amino acids. Among the 20 or more amino acids, the human body is unable to synthesize 8 and these are called essential amino acids.

The essential amino acids include:

- ✓ lysine
- ✓ tryptophan
- ✓ methionine
- ✓ leucine
- ✓ isoleucine
- ✓ phenylalanine
- ✓ valine
- ✓ threonine

Foods with the best □uality protein are eggs, milk, soybeans, meats, vegetables, and grains.

Fat In Metabolism

Fats are concentrated sources of energy. They produce twice as much energy as either carbohydrates or protein on a weight basis.

The functions of fats include:

- ✓ helping to form the cellular structure;
- ✓ forming a protective cushion and insulation around vital organs;
- ✓ helping absorb fat soluble vitamins,
- ✓ providing a reserve storage for energy

Essential fatty acids include unsaturated fatty acids like linoleic, linolinic, and arachidonic acids. These need to be taken in diet. Saturated fats, along with cholesterol, have been implicated in arteriosclerosis and heart disease.

Minerals And Vitamins In Metabolism

The minerals in foods do not contribute directly to energy needs but are important as body regulators and play a role in metabolic pathways of the body. More than 50 elements are found in the human body. About 25 elements have been found to be essential, since a deficiency produces specific deficiency symptoms.

Important minerals include:

- ✓ calcium
- ✓ phosphorus
- ✓ iron

- ✓ sodium
- ✓ potassium
- ✓ chloride ions
- ✓ copper
- ✓ cobalt
- ✓ manganese
- ✓ zinc
- ✓ magnesium
- ✓ fluorine
- ✓ iodine

Vitamins are essential organic compounds that the human body cannot synthesize by itself and must therefore, be present in the diet. Vitamins particularly important in metabolism include:

- ✓ Vitamin A
- ✓ B2 (riboflavin)
- ✓ Niacin or nicotinic acid
- ✓ Pantothenic Acid etc.

Metabolic Pathways

The chemical reactions of metabolism are organized into metabolic pathways. These allow the basic chemicals from nutrition to be transformed through a series of steps into another chemical, by a sequence of enzymes.

Enzymes are crucial to metabolism because they allow organisms to drive desirable reactions that require energy. These reactions also are coupled with those that release energy. As enzymes act as catalysts they allow these reactions to proceed quickly and efficiently. Enzymes also allow the regulation of metabolic pathways in response to changes in the cell's environment or signals from other cells.

Increasing your metabolism alone does very little for weight loss unless you combine it with other basic weight loss principles. What are those principles?

1. Drink plenty of water

Ample water is vital to weight loss and to optimum body health. For your metabolism to function at top efficiency all of your body organs and systems need adequate water. What is adequate water? Half of your body weight in ounces of water each day. In other words, if you weigh 150 pounds, you need to drink 75 ounces of water every day.

Not so-called fruit juices, soda, or coffee (especially coffee), just good, clear water. These processed fruit juices are full of sugars, flavorings, and preservatives, which are extremely detrimental to weight loss and your health in general. Coffee is nothing more than an addictive drug. It is the biggest drug habit in the world. It offers no health benefits whatsoever, in fact, it actually dehydrates your body.

2. Get 8 to 9 hours of sleep every night.
3. Cardio and weight training exercise.

It doesn't have to be body-building exercise. A light 15minute workout 2 or 3 times a day will get the job done.

1. Get out of bed, go through your first exercise session, and eat a light, healthy breakfast
2. Eat several small, healthy meals every day

Your body loves being fed good, healthy food every few hours. It hates being fed sporadically. When you feed your body sporadically, it begins storing fat because it doesn't know when it will be fed again.

So, eat all three meals. Make them light meals of carbohydrates, protein, and fiber. Stay away from the starchy carbohydrates like breads, pasta, and potatoes. Starchy carbohydrates turn to sugar in your body very quickly and your body ends up storing most of this as fat.

Eat a mid morning, mid-afternoon, and evening snack of an apple and raw nuts, or a banana and raw nuts. When you eat like this, you'll find you have no hunger pangs and you will never feel deprived of food. Your body will love it and it will stop storing fat. In fact, it will start burning fat.

Foods That Will Increase Metabolism

There are some foods that are great metabolism boosters. They act just like jet fuel in your body. They kick in your metabolism's after burner.

What are these foods?

1. **Salmon**

Salmon is one of the healthiest meats you can eat. It is a great source of monounsaturated fat and healthy protein.

2. **Turkey**

Turkey contains less fat than chicken and is very high in protein.

3. Lean, skinless chicken breast

Low in fat and high in protein

4. Broccoli

Without a doubt, the healthiest vegetable on earth

5. Whey protein shakes

Excellent source of protein and other vital nutrients

6. Apples

Great source of fiber

7. Oatmeal

Tremendous source of fiber and studies have shown it actually reduces cholesterol

8. Olives

Excellent source of monounsaturated fats

9. Beef Liver

Loaded with a ton of vitamins, minerals, and nutrients

10. Grapefruit

Lowers blood insulin levels

To receive the full benefits of these weight loss foods, make sure you consume protein, carbohydrates, and fiber with every meal, and eat small portions. Eat your healthy snacks between meals, and drink water, nothing but good, clear water.

Herbs and Spices That Will Speed Up Metabolism

1 - Garlic

Perhaps one of the most valuable and versatile foods on the planet.

2 - Ginger

Stimulates your tissues, thus using more energy and burning more calories. Ginger is also excellent for enhancing joint efficiency, reducing cholesterol, and many other health conditions.

3 - Cinnamon

Has a positive effect on blood sugar, and a great source of fiber and calcium.

4 - Cayenne Pepper

Also known as chili pepper, red pepper, and paprika. Boosts metabolism to burn fat and reduces appetite.

5 - Gensing

Boosts metabolism, energy, strength, and increases endurance.

How Metabolism Really Works

Metabolism is a process. It's the way our cells change the food we eat into the energy we need to breathe, move, think and do . . . everything. It keeps us, as it keeps all living things, alive.

Instead of being grateful for metabolism, though, we tend to blame it. No doubt you've heard someone say (or even said yourself), 'I can't lose weight. My metabolism must be slow,' "

It almost never is. Factors such as age, sex and body size cause natural variation in resting metabolic rate — the amount of calories, or units of energy, that we burn just by being alive. But those differences are normal, and they are not usually the root cause of obesity or inability to lose weight.

The real problem is almost always consuming too many calories and not getting enough exercise, which leaves us with excess energy that we store as fat. The best ways to lose weight are staying active and eating a healthy diet — not trying to change the speed of your metabolism.

But even though they can't usually increase the speed of our resting metabolic rate, our habits do affect our metabolism in five important ways:

1. How what you eat affects your metabolism

You might have heard that eating certain foods, or eating at a certain time of day, can make your metabolism faster. In reality, the speed of your metabolism remains roughly the same no matter when or what you eat. The few exceptions to this rule are not good weight loss strategies.

For example, studies have shown that caffeine slightly increases the rate at which you burn calories in the short term. But your body becomes used to caffeine over time, so the effect doesn't last if you're a regular coffee or tea drinker. Products promoted as metabolism boosters tend to be similarly ineffective, and some have dangerous side effects. So don't focus on how fast you metabolize food, but on the way you metabolize it.

That means avoiding fried foods, such as potato chips; and refined sugars, such as those found in soft drinks, candy and many baked goods. These energy sources are the most likely to end up stored as fat.

Instead, choose whole grains, lean proteins, vegetables and fruit, which your body can more readily use to fuel its functions and activities.

2. How exercise affects your metabolism

You can't do much to affect your resting metabolism, which accounts for most of the calories most people burn each day. But building muscle can help. Muscle tissue uses more energy than fat tissue does, even when you're at rest.

This is a big reason that women, who tend to have less muscle tissue than men do, also burn fewer calories. And it's why older people tend to burn fewer calories than younger people do. Loss of muscle mass is a normal part of aging, but regularly working your muscles can help combat it.

Remember, though: While building strength can boost your resting metabolism, getting more aerobic activity is the most efficient way to burn more calories. Even walking 25 or 30 minutes a day, five days a week, is helpful. And more intense exercise — running or aerobics, for example — burns even more calories.

In addition to burning calories and building muscle, exercise has been linked to increased amounts of brown fat. The vast majority of our fat is white fat, the kind that stores energy. But we also have a few ounces of brown fat, often around our neck or shoulders, which actually uses energy to help keep us warm.

3. How your current weight affects your metabolism

The process of metabolism has two main parts. Anabolism helps you grow new cells, store energy and maintain your body tissues. Catabolism breaks down fat and carbohydrate molecules to release energy that fuels anabolism, keeps you warm and enables your muscles to contract.

Insulin is one of the many hormones that help regulate this cycle, by triggering anabolism after you eat. If you're significantly overweight, there's a high risk that your body will stop responding to insulin. As a result, sugar stays in your blood instead of being stored as energy.

This is the condition we call Type 2 diabetes. It can damage your organs and put you at risk for health problems such as heart disease, stroke and kidney disease. But Type 2 diabetes isn't always permanent. Many people can reverse Type 2 diabetes by losing weight through exercise, healthier eating habits or even bariatric surgery.

4. How your former weight affects your metabolism

Having been overweight can continue to affect your metabolism even after you've lost the weight. That's one reason maintaining weight loss is much harder than keeping weight off in the first place.

Take two people who weigh the same: one who's been at a normal weight all their life, and one who has struggled with obesity: The first person can get an average amount of activity and eat an average amount of food, and nothing will happen to them. But often the second person, if they go from a restricted diet back to an average one, will have a high risk of putting a lot of the weight back on.

Researchers don't yet know exactly what causes this phenomenon. But studies have suggested that it has to do with hormonal changes after weight loss that both slow your metabolism and make you feel hungrier.

To help with this problem, doctors at Rush sometimes prescribe medications that suppress appetite. The FDA has approved a handful of appetite suppressants that have been shown to help people maintain weight loss when combined with exercise and healthy eating habits. There aren't yet medications designed to increase the speed of your metabolism.

5. How deprivation of food or sleep affects your metabolism

Regardless of your weight, eating too little can backfire by slowing the rate at which your body burns calories.

For instance, some people skip breakfast and lunch and just eat dinner. But not eating all day actually signals to your body that there's a shortage of food, so your metabolic rate goes very low. And as soon as you eat anything, your body is trying to store every single calorie in that food.

Even if you want and need to lose a lot of weight, you should aim to eat three or four small meals a day, comprising mostly vegetables, whole grains and lean proteins.

Finally, make sure you're getting seven to nine hours of sleep each night. Sleep deprivation can cause your body to produce too much insulin, which can lead to increased fat storage.

How Intermittent Fasting Work

Intermittent fasting is a controlled pattern of fasting that is made in an alternate way. Fasting? Meaning "not eat"? Yes, I really mean not to eat. Most of us when we are hungry, we chow down on foods that we can grab. This includes junk foods, processed foods and most of the time, fast foods. Anywhere we go, we see fast foods. Anywhere we go, we see street foods and so on. We eat three meals in a day and for most of us, three meals are not yet enough. We tend to feed ourselves more every time we feel the hunger or every time we feel the crave for food. We know very much that this is wrong but we do not think of it and push ourselves to give in to that craving.

Regular meals are only breakfast, lunch and dinner. These are the only meals that are important to us. Every other meal is just additional and most of the time not needed which causes us to add our weight and produce fat. When we do not work too much and physical activity is done most of the time then we might as well feed ourselves of hunger. But if we do not do physical activity much, then we should not give in to this temptous craving.

So what do we do?

This is where I can introduce intermittent fasting. This is when we eat our daily meals in a day and do fasting for the next twenty four hours. We do not necessarily mean that you cannot take in anything in your stomach. We just want you take in water or any healthy drink including fruit juice. But we recommend that water is better.

Water does a lot of good things in our body. It cleans our body and helps flush out unhealthy food. There are a lot of scientific studies and researches that proves that intermittent fasting is very beneficial to our health. Remember before that our ancestors did not have any fast foods, junk foods or street foods whenever they are hungry. What do they do? They drink water in order for their hunger to be lost. Most of the time, we feel hunger not because we really are hungry but our body and mind just dictates us to eat because it is used to. We call this mental hunger. Sometimes, our minds just cheat us.

So this is the tip on intermittent fasting. Example, today you can eat as much food as you like. But be prepared that after dinner tonight you are just allowed to drink water afterwards for twenty four hours. Drink water as much as you need to feed your hunger. This process will train your body and mind to not let you eat when you do not need to eat. This fasting will eventually lead your body to use the stored fat and energy that has not been used for a long period of time. So you will lose weight and keep you healthier.

Intermittent fasting is not advisable for all people. This is only good for individuals without health problems.

Whenever you wanted to try Intermittent fasting, you should consult first with your doctor before you push through.

Synergy With Keto

When paired with the ketogenic diet, intermittent fasting can speed up ketosis and amplify weight loss. The keto diet, which is very high in fats but low in carbs, is designed to kick-start ketosis.

Ketosis is a metabolic state that forces your body to burn fat for fuel instead of carbs. This occurs when your body is deprived of glucose, which is its main source of energy.

Combining intermittent fasting with the keto diet can help your body enter ketosis faster to maximize results. It can likewise mitigate some of the side effects that often occur when starting this diet, including the keto flu, which is characterized by nausea, headaches, and fatigue.

Intermittent Fasting is fast becoming a favored way of reducing unwanted body fat and sculpting your body the way you want it and it is not only for those gym bound health conscious fanatics that so many of the body fat burning programs are for. This works for anyone serious about reducing body fat.

For whatever the reason, be it on health grounds or purely because you want to look hotter than you do right now.

I decided to look into this a little more as it seems so many people are beginning to latch onto it, you know many of the top fitness and health experts both on and off line are now using Intermittent Fasting to help their clients lose those unwanted pounds of body fat, let me add to that - many of them are using this themselves.

<u>What better testimonial?</u>

I can now hear you saying "so tell us how does it work and is it safe" First let me answer the second element of that ᐁuestion "is it safe?"

Yes is the short and pleasing conclusion I have come to, in fact by fasting you are allowing your body the time it needs to cleanse and purify internally so not only are you losing unwanted fat and looking better on the outside but you are getting healthier internally too....how cool is that?

Back then to how it works. Intermittent Fasting is not let me repeat not starvation as many people think.

It is what it says a period of intermittent fasting; usually 24hrs at a time when you abstain from all calorific intake with the exception of water for those not clear on that (needs to be clear as I do not want to be responsible for anyone suffering unnecessarily)

During these periods of fasting you continue to maintain your existing exercise regime or if you do not have one begin one (I suggest that you speak to a fitness professional to guide you on this if you are unsure what to do).

This period of fasting should be conducted no more than 2-3 times per week with the other days consisting of a diet that is beneficial to your weight and fat loss goals (lower carbohydrates, higher protein, higher fibre) and again your exercise regime.

The days when you fast and train will ensure that your body accesses the stored body fat you are carrying for fuel/energy instead of using the calorific content of the food you are eating daily. It will burn this faster and longer on these days than the days when you eat your healthy diet.

All diets must to be effective work on the same basic principles of energy in energy out. To burn unwanted fat you must increase your activity so that you burn more calories than you store.

One other key point about the process of Intermittent fasting is the effect it has on you mind, you see for a diet to be successful you must first understand your rules about food, by fasting you are breaking the mental dependency that you have created about the food that you eat and allowing yourself to change the rules you have about food and the role it play in your life.

How Is Intermittent Fasting Riskier For Women?

Although the benefits may make you want to put down your fork immediately, not everyone will have such great results. First off, I'd recommend you talk with your doctor about IF before you try it. Ladies, IF isn't quite the same for us as it is for the guys, but I'll devote a whole section to that in a hot minute. Here's a list of people who should stay away from or get doctor's clearance before they try intermittent fasting:

- pregnant women
- people with a history of an eating disorder
- people who easily become obsessed with numbers or food
- people who are chronically stressed
- people who are diabetic (Type 1 definitely avoid, Type II- talk to Dr.)
- people who don't sleep well
- people new to healthy eating and exercise

I'm not saying intermittent fasting won't work for you – I'm saying you should talk to your doctor beforehand. Fasting creates extra stress on your body- which is actually where a lot of those cool benefits come from- but if you're already stressed, sleep deprived, or growing a human, your body won't do well with the extra stress. Fasting can have different effects on different health conditions, so involve your doctor if that applies to you. In some conditions, like IBS and Chron's, it could potentially promote the healing of your gut and reduce inflammation.

If you have a history of an eating disorder or tend to be a little OCD about things, IF, especially with counting and tracking, can easily take you down a path that will lead to further problems.

I've hinted at this throughout this guide, but felt women and IF deserved its own section. Unfortunately, not all of those benefits seem to apply to us, especially those who are using IF to lose those last 10 pounds to look cut. Remember, there just isn't enough research right now, especially on women, and we need more to tell us if it's safe or not. Some of the studies done on obese women look promising, though. Let's dive into the specifics:

❖ Mensies

Anytime a woman restricts her calories, there's a risk she will stop menstruating. Yes, this is mainly for women who are a healthy weight or on the thin side, but it's important for all women to be mindful, regardless of age or weight. Chronic stress can also cause this same thing to happen, due to stress placed on the hypothalamus, which controls our reproductive hormones. This is one reason why those who are already stressed should not proceed with IF. This stress can actually cause damage to the female hormone system, causing amenorrhea as stated above, and even early menopause (even as early as mid-20's).

Even if you don't want children, or you're not ready for them right now, missing your period is a red flag about your overall health. This includes hormones and weight gain, too. Many women report their periods stopping during IF, so this is something to watch out for. One study even found that rats' ovaries shrank while restricting calories during IF in order to divert energy to survival.

❖ **Stress**

As previously mentioned, fasting works because it places a stress on the body. This stress can cause you to burn more fat, be more alert, stay focused, and all of the other benefits mentioned. Although this seems to work great for men, women do not have the same hormonal makeup and don't appear to reap all the same benefits. One study on IF concluded female rats saw an increase in size in their adrenal glands, which signifies chronic stress during calorie restriction.

In one specific study, they tested IF and reduced calorie diets on mice. They discovered the females' brain chemistry, behavior, and hippocampus size were affected much more so than the males'. This hints that females respond more dramatically to periods of starvation and fasting than males. Women tend to have an increase in sympathetic nervous system activity during periods of fasting (which causes more alertness and anxiety), while men have more parasympathetic activity, resulting in peace and calmness. Hashtag so unfair.

❖ **Masculinizing**

Unfortunately, if you haven't noticed, this heightened response doesn't mean we reap more benefits than men. Since women respond more drastically, we can be negatively affected by the stress fasting causes, instead of improved. This is referred to as "masculinizing" (really?!) because the female rats stop menstruating, they become more alert, have better memories, and are alert/awake when they should be asleep. Many women report disrupted sleep cycles and relying heavily on coffee while intermittent fasting.

❖ Glucose and Insulin

Women also don't seem to reap the same benefits of increased insulin resistance or glucose tolerance. One study showed women experienced a decrease in glucose tolerance. This means IF actually harmed women's metabolism, not boosted, and moved them toward a pre-diabetic state. On the other hand, a pro is that women experienced an increase in good cholesterol (HDL) in this study on ADF while men did not. Before you get too excited, these women also experienced increased ghrelin, which is a hunger arousing hormone.

❖ Energy

At first this anxiety and alertness can seem beneficial and people get more done; the long-term effects of this are negative, and many women report this "energy" is short-lived. By contrast, others feel such low energy they significantly increase the amount of coffee they drink, which can also wreak havoc on hormones and be especially harmful to those who don't have the coffee gene.

To me, these risks outweigh the potential pros of IF for women. Although both you and I know women who've experienced great results with IF, the research presents more reason for ladies to be cautious and hesitant than gung ho about shortening our eating windows.

CHAPTER TWO

INTERMITTENT FASTING MYTHS

No matter what type of eating plan you start, there will always be criticizers who call it too tough or harmful. That's why it's important to have all the information before you begin and to debunk many common myths. We're taking some of the common myths about intermittent fasting and debunking them below

1. Think You'll Starve to Death!

You are going to feel hungry at first as your body adjusts to a longer period without food – that's only natural. But, having your body adapt to change in diet is what causes physical changes like weight loss and health benefits. There is a stark difference in going without needed nutrition and choosing not to eat during a specific time period while still eating when needed. When you're deciding to fast, you're voluntarily restricting your calories, and you have the reassurance that at the end of your fasting window you will be able to eat. Intermittent fasting is all about timing. By extending the amount of time you are going without food, your body's hormones and metabolism begin to change in order to encourage weight loss.

2. Small Meals Are Essential

They're not. Intermittent fasting is about the quality of calories you're taking in when you are eating so that you can make it through the fasting window. When you are eating a diet with enough calories, you then have the energy to last through the fasting period and will not need to have a snack or a meal. Eating some small meals might help you feel better in the short term, as they soothe your growling stomach, but it won't help you gain the health benefits of fasting or spur on weight loss. It could do the opposite and increase your caloric intake and have your weight loss stop. That only helps when you extend your window of time without food and allow your body to burn fat it has stored away.

3. But Humans Can't Survive Without Water!

This is 100% true, and that's why when you are fasting, you are encouraged to up your water intake, so you don't become dehydrated. If you want to fast for a long period of time, having enough water will help you do that, and other beverages like coffee or tea will give you a more filling effect. If plain water isn't enough for you, try infusing your ice cubes with some low-calorie fruit or mint in order to give your water more flavor. Remember, you can also have beverages so long as you are not taking them with cream or artificial sweeteners. Those "empty calories" might seem like nothing but believe me they can add up.

4.   Your Brain Will Be Starved of Glucose

Many people are misguided in the belief that your brain will be deprived of glucose when you fast, but once again, that just isn't true. Your brain does need glucose, but a window of time without food doesn't mean your brain will be deprived of energy. When you skip a meal and are not having an intake of carbohydrates, your brain will get energy from ketones of fat molecules instead of glucose from carbohydrates. They are a great energy-rich fuel, and studies show that they actually improve cognitive functioning.

5.   I'll Lose My Hard-Gained Muscle

I was concerned about this but there is no need to be. This is another myth where people think that participating in intermittent fasting will suddenly cause your muscles to shrink and disappear. That's just not true. After you eat a meal, your body is working hard to break down that food into molecules it uses for energy. It processes proteins, fats, and carbohydrates to store away. After it's used the meal for fuel, what will it do for more energy if you've decided to skip your next meal? We can assure you it doesn't turn on your muscles. It will instead turn to fat reserves it has stored away as energy and uses those to power you through the day.

A fasting window of anywhere from 12 to 20 hours is not enough time for an athlete to lose their muscles. The general rule of thumb is that fasting for a period of 48 hours or longer can be harmful. But, a short span of missing a meal or two does not have detrimental effects on the body's muscle mass.

Another truth that discounts this myth is that it takes a long time for the protein to be fully digested and absorbed by the body. It takes your body approximately six hours to burn off the protein of three eggs at the rate of 2.9 grams of protein an hour. If you drink a protein shake with twenty-six grams of soy protein powder, then it will take you approximately seven hours to absorb the protein at a rate of 3.9 an hour. Different protein sources are absorbed at different rates, between 1 and 10 grams of protein an hour depending on the source. As you can see, if you eat a large amount of protein before your fast, it can fuel you through either all or more of your entire fast!

6.   Small Meals Increase Metabolism

This is a common myth, that is again, not true. People believe that the more you eat during the day; your metabolism will increase with each small meal. Yes, your body must expend more energy to digest every small meal that you're eating, but that energy depends on the total calories you eat, not how many times a day you eat. So, eating 4 different three-hundred calorie meals will expend the same energy as eating two six-hundred calorie meals. The frequency of your meals will not impact how many calories you burn.

The only way you will be calorie deficient enough to actually lose weight is by taking in fewer calories than you are expanding. By eating less and including exercise in your diet, your body will need to burn fat for energy to keep up with you. That's when real weight loss occurs. If you're stuffing yourself with empty calories throughout the day, your blood sugar will rise each time, and that can lead to more health conditions.

7. I'll Binge Like Crazy After Fasting and Gain Weight

If you do intermittent fasting properly, you won't gain weight. This is only true if you overeat when you aren't fasting. It all depends on your individual behavior. You just need to get used to the fasting routine, and your appetite may even diminish as you continue with it. To help yourself not binge eat after you finish fasting, you can practice by starting your fast gradually. Don't immediately jump into a sixteen-hour fast. Instead, try skipping a meal when you are naturally not hungry or doing an overnight twelve-hour fast between dinner and breakfast.

Non-fasting calories just need to stay below the calories missed while fasting for you to lose weight. The key is to eat healthy filling meals when you aren't fasting, not ones that are loaded with unhealthy ingredients and excessive calories. Sure, you might end up eating a few hundred calories more to compensate for the "lost" calories during your fasting window, but that overeating amount is still less than what you would have eaten for a full day without fasting.

8. Protein is Only Needed in Small Doses Throughout the Day for Muscle Growth

This is another common myth that science has debunked. It used to be that athletes believed they had to constantly supply their body with protein throughout the day for their muscles to continue to grow after a workout. New, research has shown that muscle growth actually occurs in the hours after you work out. Eating protein throughout the day won't increase your muscle growth.

You simply need to eat your recommended amount of protein during the hours you are not fasting. This could even be all in one meal, but it is usually easier to stagger your protein intake over a time frame. It's a bit easier on your stomach too.

9. Twelve Hours without Food is far too Long. I Might Pass Out or Try to Eat My Arm!

When you see the number as individual hours, it can seem like a very long time and very hard to do. But the truth is, you might be fasting for twelve hours without even realizing it. Let's say you have dinner at seven in the evening and are strict with yourself about no snacking before bed. Then the next morning, you're busy with getting ready and getting the kids to school that you have a cup of coffee but don't have breakfast until almost seven. That means you've fasted twelve hours without even realizing it It's all about structuring your day around your individual schedule. For sixteen hours, you would bump up your breakfast time to more of a brunch time. Treat yourself to enough coffee and water or tea to keep yourself going, and then have your first meal around eleven in the morning. That's a sixteen hour fast. This a great method to get you started.

10. I'm Concerned that Fasting will Affect my Athletic Performance!

Another common myth is that fasting will hurt athletes in their performance on the field or in their workouts. Yet, research shows that this is not true. Intermittent fasting does not interfere with your body's performance when done correctly. Sure, when you start your fasting period, you might feel weak or slow, but that's because your body is simply adjusting to the change. It would be the same way if you started a new diet plan or cut caffeine or sugar from your diet. Once your body realizes you're not eating a meal for energy, it begins to burn the fat molecules it has stored away for energy. With that burst of energy, you can exercise, train, and play just like you normally would. Keep in mind, intermittent fasting recommends a higher intake of water as well, so that there is no risk of dehydration.

11. Fasting May Damage my Overall Health

There's no way on Earth that I would do that to my body. We understand that the first conclusion people will assume about not eating is that your body is in trouble. Although, the science proves otherwise. Research and studies show that intermittent fasting has a variety of health benefits as were as discussing. Weight loss is an obvious physical result, but it can also control your blood sugar, lower your cholesterol, and give you higher mental functioning and clarity. As with any change in your diet, it's important you speak to your doctor first to make sure you're a healthy candidate to follow an intermittent fasting model and that you would not be harming your health.

We've provided you the truth when it comes to these common myths about intermittent fasting so you are informed about how fasting will affect you.

CHAPTER THREE

TYPES OF INTERMTTENT FASTING

Intermittent fasting comes in various forms and each may have a specific set of uni□ue benefits. Each form of intermittent fasting has variations in the fasting-to-eating ratio. The benefits and effectiveness of these different protocols may differ on an individual basis and it is important to determine which one is best for you. Factors that may influence which one to choose include health goals, daily schedule/routine, and current health status. The most common types of IF are alternate day fasting, time-restricted feeding, and modified fasting.

1) MODIFIED FASTING - 5:2 DIET

Modified fasting is a protocol with programmed fasting days, but the fasting days do allow for some food intake. Generally, 20-25% of normal calories are allowed to be consumed on fasting days; so if you normally consume 2000 calories on regular eating days, you would be allowed 400-500 calories on fasting days. The 5:2 part of this diet refers to the ratio of non-fasting to fasting days.

So on this regimen you would eat normally for 5 consecutive days, then fast or restrict calories to 20-25% for 2 consecutive days.

This protocol is great for weight loss, body composition, and may also benefit the regulation of blood sugar, lipids, and inflammation. Studies have shown the 5:2 protocol to be effective for weight loss, improve/lower inflammation markers in the blood, and show signs trending improvements in insulin resistance. In animal studies, this modified fasting 5:2 diet resulted in decreased fat, decreased hunger hormones (leptin), and increased levels of a protein responsible for improvements in fat burning and blood sugar regulation (adiponectin).

The modified 5:2 fasting protocol is easy to follow and has a small number of negative side effects which included hunger, low energy, and some irritability when beginning the program. Contrary to this however, studies have also noted improvements such as reduced tension, less anger, less fatigue, improvements in self confidence, and a more positive mood.

2) TIME-RESTRICTED FEEDING:

If you know anyone that has said they are doing intermittent fasting, odds are it is in the form of time-restricted feeding. This is a type of intermittent fasting that is used daily and it involves only consuming calories during a small portion of the day and fasting for the remainder. Daily fasting intervals in time-restricted feeding may range from 12-20 hours, with the most common method being 16/8 (fasting for 16 hours, consuming calories for 8). For this protocol the time of day is not important as long as you are fasting for a consecutive period of time and only eating in your allowed time period. For example, on a 16/8 time-restricted feeding program one person may eat their first meal at 7AM and last meal at 3PM (fast from 3PM-7AM), while another person may eat their first meal at 1PM and last meal at 9PM (fast from 9PM-1PM). This protocol is meant to be performed every day over long periods of time and is very flexible as long as you are staying within the fasting/eating window(s).

Time-Restricted feeding is one of the most easy to follow methods of intermittent fasting. Using this along with your daily work and sleep schedule may help achieve optimal metabolic function. Time-restricted feeding is a great program to follow for weight loss and body composition improvements as well as some other overall health benefits. The few human trials that were conducted noted significant reductions in weight, reductions in fasting blood glucose, and improvements in cholesterol with no changes in perceived tension, depression, anger, fatigue, or confusion. Some other preliminary results from animal studies showed time restricted feeding to protect against obesity, high insulin levels, fatty liver disease, and inflammation.

The easy application and promising results of time-restricted feeding could possibly make it an excellent option for weight loss and chronic disease prevention/management. When implementing this protocol it may be good to begin with a lower fasting-to-eating ratio like 12/12 hours and eventually work your way up to 16/8 hours.

3) The 16/8 Method: Fast for 16 hours each day.

The 16/8 Method involves fasting every day for 14-16 hours, and restricting your daily "eating window" to 8-10 hours.

Doing this method of fasting can actually be as simple as not eating anything after dinner, and skipping breakfast. For example, if you finish your last meal at 8 pm and then don't eat until 12 noon the next day, then you are technically fasting for 16 hours between meals.

It is generally recommended that women only fast 14-15 hours, because they seem to do better with slightly shorter fasts. For people who get hungry in the morning and like to eat breakfast, then this can be hard to get used to at first. However, many breakfast skippers actually instinctively eat this way.

You can drink water, coffee and other non-caloric beverages during the fast, and this can help reduce hunger levels. It is very important to eat mostly healthy foods during your eating window. This won't work if you eat lots of junk food or excessive amounts of calories.

4) Eat-Stop-Eat:

Eat-Stop-Eat involves a 24-hour fast, either once or twice per week. By fasting from dinner one day, to dinner the next, this amounts to a 24-hour fast.

For example, if you finish dinner on Monday at 7 pm, and don't eat until dinner the next day at 7 pm, then you've just done a full 24-hour fast. You can also fast from breakfast to breakfast, or lunch to lunch. The end result is the same. Water, coffee and other non-caloric beverages are allowed during the fast, but no solid food.

If you are doing this to lose weight, then it is very important that you eat normally during the eating periods. As in, eat the same amount of food as if you hadn't been fasting at all. The problem with this method is that a full 24-hour fast can be fairly difficult for many people.

However, you don't need to go all-in right away, starting with 14-16 hours and then moving upwards from there is fine.

5) Alternate-Day Fasting:

Alternate-Day fasting means fasting every other day. There are several different versions of this. Some of them allow about 500 calories during the fasting days. Many of the lab studies showing health benefits of intermittent fasting used some version of this.

A full fast every other day seems rather extreme, so I do not recommend this for beginners. With this method, you will be going to bed very hungry several times per week, which is not very pleasant and probably unsustainable in the long-term.

6) Spontaneous Meal Skipping:

You don't actually need to follow a structured intermittent fasting plan to reap some of the benefits. Another option is to simply skip meals from time to time, when you don't feel hungry or are too busy to cook and eat. It is a myth that people need to eat every few hours or they will hit "starvation mode" or lose muscle.

The human body is well equipped to handle long periods of famine, let alone missing one or two meals from time to time. So if you're really not hungry one day, skip breakfast and just eat a healthy lunch and dinner. Or if you're travelling somewhere and can't find anything you want to eat, do a short fast. Skipping 1 or 2 meals when you feel so inclined is basically a spontaneous intermittent fast. Just make sure to eat healthy foods at the other meals.

7) The Warrior Diet:

It involves eating small amounts of raw fruits and vegetables during the day, then eating one huge meal at night. Basically, you "fast" all day and "feast" at night within a 4 hour eating window. The Warrior Diet was one of the first popular "diets" to include a form of intermittent fasting. This diet also emphasizes food choices that are quite similar to a paleo diet - whole, unprocessed foods that resemble what they looked like in nature.

8) 20/4 Method

Unlike the Warrior Diet briefly described above, the 20:4 Intermittent Fasting protocol used by the low-carb community today alternates a lengthy fasting period with a traditional ketogenic diet. The lengthy fast allows insulin to stay low for an extended period of time.

The "20" in the 20:4 formula means you go 20 hours without eating anything, including ketogenic foods.

- ✓ All you can have is no-calorie liquids.
- ✓ This isn't as bad as it sounds because you'll be sleeping for 8 of those 20 hours.
- ✓ The 20 hour fast is called the fasting window.
- ✓ The "4" in the 20:4 formula means you eat a normal keto diet during the four consecutive hours that you're not fasting.

✓ The 4 hour eating period is called the eating window.

<u>The hours you eat is up to you.</u>

You don't have to limit your eating to just evenings. You can tailor your 20 hours of fasting and 4-hour eating window to fit your personal preferences, hunger level, and what's going on in your life.

This is where things get really difficult, and every day becomes a test of willpower and mental fortitude. Doing a 20:4 intermittent fasting schedule is extremely tough, and most people will have difficulty sticking to this on a consistent basis.

With a mere 4-hour eating window, you barely have enough time to get two meals in. Most people will have one big meal and then snack the rest of the way. Fasting for 20 hours means you have your first meal at around 4 o'clock in the evening, just before you clock out of work, and finish eating by 8.

It's a truly short period of time for most people, and only the absolutely dedicated intermittent fasting practitioners can do it.

CHAPTER FOUR

WHAT TO EAT WHILE INTERMITTENT FASTING

Eating during intermittent fasting (IF) can be confusing. This is because IF is not a diet plan but an eating pattern. Keeping this in mind, experts at DoFasting have created an intermittent fasting food list that will keep you healthy while you are on your weight loss journey.

IF tells you about when to eat but does not mention what foods can be included in your diet. A lack of clear dietary guidelines can give a false impression that one can eat whatever they want. For others, this can cause problems with choosing the "right" foods and drinks.

These not only sabotage your weight-loss efforts but can also make you more likely to be undernourished or overnourished.

There are many ways to do intermittent fasting. Some of them are:

– 5:2 FAST

This flexible method of fasting is popular among beginners. In this method, you can eat normally for five days each week. During the remaining 2 days, you should limit your daily calorie intake to about 500 calories.

– 12-HOUR FAST

Like the 5:2 fast, this is another beginner-friendly fasting method. It is easy to follow. Simply, avoid eating any calories for 12 hours. Eat all your calories within the next 12 hours. That completes one cycle of fasting.

Once your body adapts to fasting for 12 hours, you can work your way up to fasting for longer durations, such as the 16:8 fast or 20-hour fast.

– 16-HOUR FAST

This is probably the most studied form of IF. We may say it is an extended version of the 12-hour fast. You are not allowed to eat for 16 hours a day and can eat normally in the 8-hour feeding window. Want more information

<u>Intermittent Fasting Food List: How to Choose the Best Foods</u>

Eating during intermittent fasting is more about being healthy than just rapidly losing your weight. Thus, it is critically important to choose nutrient-dense foods such as veggies, fruits, lean proteins, and healthy fats.

The intermittent fasting food list should contain:

1. For Protein

The Recommended Dietary Allowance (RDA) for protein is 0.8 grams of protein per kilogram of body weight. Your requirements may vary depending on your fitness goals and level of activity.

Protein helps you lose weight by decreasing energy intake, increasing satiety, and boosting metabolism.

Besides, when combined with strength training, increased protein intake helps build muscle. Having more muscle in the body naturally increases your metabolism, as muscle burns more calories than fat. A recent study suggests that having more muscle in your legs can help reduce belly fat formation in healthy men.

The IF food list for protein include:

- ✓ Poultry and fish
- ✓ Eggs

✓ Seafood

✓ Dairy products such as milk, yogurt, and cheese

✓ Seeds and nuts

✓ Beans and legumes

✓ Soy

✓ Whole grains

2. FOR CARBS

According to the Dietary Guidelines for Americans, 45 to 65 percent of your daily calories should come from carbohydrates (carbs). Carbs are the major source of energy for your body. The other two are protein and fat. Carbs come in various forms. The most notable of them are sugar, fiber, and starch.

Carbs often get a bad rap for causing weight gain. However, not all carbs are created equal and they are not inherently fattening. Whether or not you will gain weight depends on the type and quantity of the carbs you eat. Make sure to choose foods that are high in fiber and starch but low in sugar.

A 2015 study suggests that eating 30 grams of fiber each day can cause weight loss, improve glucose levels, and lower blood pressure. Getting 30 grams of fiber from your diet is not an uphill challenge. You can get them by eating a simple egg sandwich, Mediterranean barley with chickpeas, apple with peanut butter, and chicken and black peas enchiladas.

The IF food list for carbs include:

- ✓ Sweet potatoes
- ✓ Beetroots
- ✓ Quinoa
- ✓ Oats
- ✓ Brown rice
- ✓ Bananas
- ✓ Mangoes
- ✓ Apples
- ✓ Berries
- ✓ Kidney beans
- ✓ Pears
- ✓ Avocado
- ✓ Carrots
- ✓ Broccoli
- ✓ Brussels sprouts
- ✓ Almonds
- ✓ Chia seeds

✓ Chickpeas

3. FOR FATS

According to the 2015-2020 Dietary Guidelines for Americans, fats should contribute 20% to 35% of your daily calories. Most notably, saturated fat should not contribute more than 10% of daily calories. Fats can be good, bad, or simply in-between depending on the type.

For example, trans fats increase inflammation, reduce the levels of the "good" cholesterol, and increase the levels of the "bad" cholesterol. They are found in fried foods and baked goods. Saturated fats can increase the risk of heart disease. However, expert opinions differ on this. It's wise to eat them in moderation. Red meat, whole milk, coconut oil, and baked goods contain high amounts of saturated fats.

Healthy fats include monounsaturated and polyunsaturated fats. These fats can reduce the risk of heart disease, lower blood pressure, and reduce the blood levels of fats.

Olive oil, peanut oil, canola oil, safflower oil, sunflower oil, and soybean oils are rich sources of these fats.

The IF food list for fats include:

- ✓ Avocados
- ✓ Nuts
- ✓ Cheese
- ✓ Whole eggs
- ✓ Dark chocolate
- ✓ Fatty fish
- ✓ Chia seeds
- ✓ Extra virgin olive oil (EVOO)
- ✓ Full-fat yogurt

4. FOR A HEALTHY GUT

A growing body of evidence shows that your gut health is the key to your overall health. Your gut is home to billions of bacteria known as the microbiota. These bacteria affect your gut health, digestion, and mental health. They may also play a crucial role in many chronic disorders.

Thus, you should take care of those tiny bugs in your stomach, especially when you are intermittent fasting.

The intermittent fasting food list for a healthy gut include:

- ✓ All vegetables
- ✓ Fermented vegetables
- ✓ Kefir
- ✓ Kimchi
- ✓ Kombucha
- ✓ Miso
- ✓ Sauerkraut
- ✓ Tempeh

In addition to keeping your gut healthy, these foods can also help you lose weight by:

- Decreasing the absorption of fat from the gut.
- Increasing the excretion of ingested fat through stools.
- Reducing food intake.

5. FOR HYDRATION

According to the National Academies of Sciences, Engineering, and Medicine, the daily fluid requirement is:

- About 15.5 cups (3.7 liters) for men.
- About 11.5 cups (2.7 liters) for women.
- Fluids include water as well as foods and drinks that contain water.

Staying hydrated during intermittent fasting is critical to your health. Dehydration can cause headaches, extreme tiredness, and dizziness. If you are already struggling with these side effects of fasting, dehydration can make them worse or even serious.

The intermittent fasting food list for hydration include:

- ✓ Water
- ✓ Sparkling water
- ✓ Black coffee or tea
- ✓ Watermelon
- ✓ Strawberries
- ✓ Cantaloupe
- ✓ Peaches
- ✓ Oranges

- ✓ Skim milk
- ✓ Lettuce
- ✓ Cucumber
- ✓ Celery
- ✓ Tomatoes
- ✓ Plain yogurt

Interestingly, taking plenty of water can also help with weight loss. A 2016 review study states that proper hydration can help you lose weight by:

- ✓ Decreasing appetite or food intake.
- ✓ Increasing fat burning.
- ✓ Foods to Exclude from the Intermittent Fasting Food List
- ✓ Processed foods
- ✓ Refined grains
- ✓ Trans-fat
- ✓ Sugar-sweetened beverages
- ✓ Candy bars
- ✓ Processed meat
- ✓ Alcoholic beverages

<u>Combining Intermittent Fasting with Specific Diets: Things to Know</u>

Some people believe that combining IF with certain diets such as the keto diet or a vegetarian diet is more effective for weight loss. That said, the jury is still out on whether or not this is true. Want to try the combination of IF and the keto diet? Make sure to include the following in the high-fat low carb diet intermittent fasting food list:

FOR FATS (75% OF YOUR DAILY CALORIES)

- ✓ Avocados
- ✓ Nuts
- ✓ Cheese
- ✓ Whole eggs
- ✓ Dark chocolate
- ✓ Fatty fish
- ✓ Chia seeds
- ✓ Extra virgin olive oil (EVOO)
- ✓ Full-fat yogurt

FOR PROTEIN (20% OF YOUR DAILY CALORIES)

- ✓ Poultry and fish
- ✓ Eggs
- ✓ Seafood
- ✓ Dairy products such as milk, yogurt, and cheese

✓ Seeds and nuts

✓ Beans and legumes

✓ Soy

✓ Whole grains

FOR CARBS (5% OF YOUR DAILY CALORIES)

✓ Sweet potatoes

✓ Beetroots

✓ Quinoa

✓ Oats

✓ Brown rice

The food list for intermittent fasting vegetarian diet includes:

– FOR PROTEIN

- Dairy products such as milk, yogurt, and cheese
- Seeds and nuts
- Beans and legumes
- Soy
- Whole grains

– FOR CARBS

- Sweet potatoes
- Beetroots

- Quinoa
- Oats
- Brown rice
- Bananas
- Mangoes
- Apples
- Berries
- Kidney beans
- Pears
- Avocado
- Carrots
- Broccoli
- Brussels sprouts
- Almonds
- Chia seeds
- Chickpeas

– FOR FATS

- Avocados
- Nuts
- Cheese
- Dark chocolate
- Chia seeds

- Extra virgin olive oil (EVOO)
- Full-fat yogurt

Intermittent fasting is one of the most studied tools for healthy weight loss.

Eating foods such as veggies, nuts, seeds, lean proteins, and fruits can enhance the weight loss benefits of intermittent fasting. Healthy eating during intermittent fasting is the key to preventing nutritional deficiencies.

You can combine fasting with popular diets such as the keto diet or a vegetarian diet.

CHAPTER FIVE

20 EASY HEALTHY RECIPES

1. Easy Shrimp & Avocado Salad with Seafood Sauce

This salad is so fresh and tasty and can be pulled together in just a few minutes. Featuring delicious shrimp paired with creamy avocado, you can't ask for a healthier lunch or dinner.

Topped with the easiest seafood sauce you'll ever make? It's pure heaven. Enjoy this easy, Whole30 compliant salad made with shrimp, avocado and dressing made with heart-healthy fats.

Ingredients (makes 4 servings)

Salad:

- ✓ 500 g cooked and peeled shrimp (1.1 lb)
- ✓ 2 small gem lettuces (200 g/ 7.1 oz)
- ✓ 1 large avocado (200 g/ 7.1 oz)
- ✓ 1 tbsp chopped cilantro (coriander)
- ✓ 1 tbsp lemon juice (15 ml)

✓ sea salt and ground pepper, to taste

Seafood Sauce:

- ✓ 1/2 cup paleo mayonnaise (110 g/ 3.9 oz) - you can make your own mayo
- ✓ 2 tbsp sugar-free ketchup (30 g/ 1.1 oz) - you can make your own ketchup
- ✓ 1 tsp Worcestershire sauce or coconut aminos
- ✓ pinch of cayenne pepper, to taste

Instructions

1. Prepare all the ingredients.
2. Place all of the sauce ingredients into a small bowl and whisk until smooth and well combined. Pour into a serving bowl or jug.
3. Season the shrimp with salt and pepper. Peel and slice the avocado and toss the slices in the lemon juice to stop browning.
4. Tear the lettuce into chunks and spread out on a serving tray or bowl. Scatter the shrimp all around the lettuce and then tuck the avocado slices amongst the shrimp. (Note: For better portion control, divide between 4 small single-serve salad bowls.)

5. Finish with a scatter of coriander (cilantro). Serve with lemon wedges, if desired. Store in a covered container in the fridge for up to 3 days.

2. Low-Carb Green Eggs with Smoked Salmon

Don't let a busy morning stop you from having a delicious breakfast. If you're hungry but barely have 10 minutes, make these simple low-carb green eggs and salmon in just 5 minutes!

A simple meal made with whole foods combined with intermittent fasting is the best way to keep keto eating effortless and easy to follow in the long run. I usually eat just two meals per day so this would either be my breakfast, brunch or lunch.

Ingredients (makes 1 serving)

- ✓ 100 g frozen spinach, thawed and drained (3.5 oz)
- ✓ 1 tbsp ghee, lard or duck fat (15 ml)
- ✓ 3 large eggs
- ✓ sea salt and ground black pepper, to taste
- ✓ 3 slices smoked salmon (85 g/ 3 oz)
- ✓ 1 tbsp chopped chives or spring onion

✓ 1 tbsp extra virgin olive oil (15 ml)

Instructions

1. S☐ueeze out all the excess water from the spinach. (You should end up with just about 43 g/ 1.5 oz drained spinach per serving.)Low-Carb Green Eggs with Smoked Salmon

2. In a bowl, lightly beat the eggs with salt and pepper until just combined. Chop the drained spinach and set aside.Low-Carb Green Eggs with Smoked Salmon

3. Pour in the eggs and swirl the pan to coat the bottom. Using a wooden spoon or a rubber spatula, gently push the edges into the middle of the pan. The uncooked runny eggs should spill out and coat the base of the pan.

4. After just about a minute, add the chopped spinach. Cook until the eggs are just set, and then remove from heat.

5. To serve, place the eggs on a plate and add the smoked salmon. Sprinkle with chives and drizzle with olive oil. Serve immediately.

3. Easy Full English Keto Breakfast

This recipe is my healthier version of a popular British all-day breakfast meal. I skipped the commonly used baked beans in sweet tomato sauce, potato hash browns, black pudding and sausages (although you could always add gluten-free sausages!). Instead I added sliced avocado for healthy fats and potassium, spinach for magnesium, roasted mushrooms and sweet cherry tomatoes. This is a great way to get all the nutrients you need in one delicious meal that takes 15 minutes to prepare!

There is a simple rule you need to follow if you want to try intermittent fasting: You'll need to make your portions more satisfying which meant that you need to worry less about eating too many calories and more about eating enough nutrient-dense foods. This means more protein, more fat and also more calories per meal. For those who regularly practice intermittent fasting, it's not uncommon to eat over 1,000 calories in just one meal.

Ingredients (makes 1 serving)

- ✓ 1 tbsp ghee, lard or duck fat (15 ml)

- ✓ 4 to 5 brown mushrooms or 1 large Portobello mushroom (85 g/ 3 oz)
- ✓ 5-6 thin-cut or 2-3 regular slices bacon (75 g/ 2.7 oz)
- ✓ 2 large eggs
- ✓ 1/2 cup frozen and thawed spinach (78 g/ 2.8 oz), excess juices drained
- ✓ 4-5 cherry tomatoes on the vine (40 g/ 1.4 oz)
- ✓ 1/2 medium avocado, sliced (75 g/ 2.7 oz)
- ✓ salt, pepper and/or chili pepper flakes to taste

Optional: 1 to 2 gluten-free Italian sausages for extra protein, plus 1 tbsp extra virgin olive oil for extra fats to drizzle on top

Instructions

1. Heat a skillet greased with ghee over a medium-high heat. Cook the mushrooms seasoned with salt and pepper, top side down, for about 5 minutes. Flip and cook for about 2 more minutes until they are tender. Transfer to a plate.

2. Fry the bacon until crispy. Fry the eggs until the white is cooked through and opaque, and the yolk is still runny. Tilt the skillet and pour the hot oil over the egg white to help it cook faster.

3. Place the cherry tomatoes in the pan where you cooked the bacon and egg and fry on high for just about a minute. Frying is optional and you can serve the tomatoes fresh if you prefer that.

4. Drain the spinach (once you squeeze out the water, you'll get about 40% of the original weight, about 30 g/ 1 oz drained sspinach). Optionally, throw in the pan where you cooked the egg to heat through.

5. Serve everything with sliced avocado. Season to taste and enjoy immediately.

4. Low-Carb Breakfast Burrito

Ingredients (makes 2 burritos)

- ✓ 2 homemade Keto Tortillas (each 8-inch/ 20 cm)
- ✓ 1/2 cup Quick Tomato Salsa (120 g/ 4.2 oz)
- ✓ 3 large eggs
- ✓ 1 tbsp unsweetened almond milk (15 ml)
- ✓ pinch sea salt and pepper
- ✓ 1 tbsp ghee, butter or olive oil for frying (15 ml)
- ✓ 3 tbsp sour cream (45 ml)
- ✓ 1/2 cup grated cheddar cheese (57 g/ 2 oz)

✓ 1/2 large avocado, thinly sliced (100 g/ 3.5 oz)

Instructions

1. Prepare the Keto Tortillas (or use store bought low-carb tortillas, beware of the ingredients used), and the Quick Tomato Salsa Making both from scratch will take an extra hour to prepare but can be made in advance. It then takes less than 15 minutes to assemble.

2. To scramble the eggs, add to a small bowl and whisk with the almond milk. Season with salt and pepper.

3. Add the oil to a medium-sized fry pan over low to medium heat. Add the eggs and cook, stirring gently and occasionally with a wooden spoon until just cooked.

4. To assemble, place the tortillas on two plates and top with the cheese.

5. Place the scrambled eggs on top – this will begin to melt the cheese slightly. Top with the avocado, salsa and sour cream.

6. Roll up and serve immediately.

5. The Best Low-Carb Eggplant Lasagna

If you follow a vegan keto diet, it will be a bit more challenging to find healthy alternatives while keeping the carbs low. You could swap the cheese layer and the mozzarella for almond-based dairy alternatives and instead of the ghee, simply use coconut oil or olive oil. You could swap the parmesan for nutritional yeast. Skip the egg omelettes — as used in my Vegetarian Keto Lasagna — and use more veggies instead.

Ingredients (makes 4 servings)

- ✓ 2 medium eggplants, sliced into 1/2 inch (1 cm) slices (500 g/ 1.1 lb)
- ✓ 2 tbsp melted ghee or duck fat, divided (30 ml)
- ✓ 1/2 medium yellow onion (50 g/ 1.8 oz)
- ✓ 500 g ground beef (1.1 lb)
- ✓ 1/3 cup sugar-free marinara sauce (80 ml/ 2.7 fl oz) - you can make your own Marinara Sauce
- ✓ 1 cup ricotta cheese (240 g/ 8.5 oz)
- ✓ 2 tbsp chopped parsley
- ✓ 2 tbsp chopped mint
- ✓ sea salt and black pepper, to taste
- ✓ 1 large egg

- ✓ 3/4 cup + 2 tbsp grated mozzarella cheese (100 g/ 3.5 oz)
- ✓ 2/3 cup grated Parmesan cheese (60 g/ 2.1 oz)

Instructions

1. Brush the eggplant slices with 1 tablespoon of ghee from both sides. Place in the oven and bake at 200 °C/ 400 °F (fan assisted), or 220 °C/ 425 °F (conventional) for 20 minutes.
2. Remove from the oven and set aside to cool.
3. Grease a pan with 1 tablespoon of ghee and cook the onion for a few minutes until fragrant. Add the beef and cook until browned and opaque.
4. Add marinara sauce and mix (reserve about a tablespoon for later). Take off the heat.
5. In a bowl, mix the ricotta, chopped herbs, salt, pepper, and egg. Mix until well combined and creamy.
6. Spread the remaining marinara sauce in the baking tray. We used a 12.5 x 10 inch (32 x 26 cm) baking dish per 4 servings, but any large deep dish will work. Add a third of the roasted eggplant slices. You'll be making three layers of eggplant in total.

7. Spread half of the ricotta mixture over them and add half of the cooked beef. Repeat one more time and finally add the last layer of eggplant slices.

8. Top with grated mozzarella and Parmesan. Bake in the oven preheated to 180 °C/ 360 °F (fan) for 30 minutes.

9. Let it cool down slightly before serving. You can store the cooled low-carb lasagne in the fridge for up to 4 days. Freezing is not recommended as it will change the texture of the cheese layer.

6. Keto Bacon Wrapped Chicken Parcels

These delightful parcels of tender and moist chicken, filled with herby cheese and wrapped in crispy bacon, these simple chicken parcels is what you need in your life. The hardest part is waiting for the filling to chill, but trust me, this is crucial to stopping the cheese simply oozing out and being wasted.

Ingredients (makes 4 servings)

- ✓ 4 medium chicken breasts (800 kg/ 1.76 lb)
- ✓ cream cheese (200 g/ 7.1 oz)
- ✓ 1/2 cup grated Parmesan cheese or hard cheese of choice (45 g/ 1.6 oz)

- ✓ 2 tbsp chopped parsley or herbs of choice
- ✓ sea salt and pepper, to taste
- ✓ 8 thin-cut slices of bacon or 4 regular slices halved widthwise (120 g/ 4.2 oz)

Instructions

1. Start by preparing the cheese stuffing.
2. Place the cream cheese, parmesan and parsley together in a bowl and beat well to combine. Divide into four and, using cling wrap, roll into logs the length of your chicken. Place in the freezer until frozen, approx. half an hour.
3. Preheat oven to 200 °C/ 400 °F (fan assisted), or 220 °C/ 425 °F (conventional). Line a baking tray. Place the chicken on the tray and cut a pocket into the top of each one. Don't cut all of the way through, just pocket for your cheese. Place the frozen cream cheese mixture into each one.
4. Wrap each breast in two slices of thin bacon, securing with a toothpick if necessary. Bake for 30 minutes.
5. Broil for an additional 2 minutes if the bacon needs crisping up. Store, wrapped in cling wrap, in the fridge for up to 4 days.

7. **Quick Keto Salmon Power Bowl**

Sometimes the really simple recipes are the best. I love how throwing a healthy ingredients that you have on hand together can create a really wholesome, flavourful keto-approved and diabetic-friendly meal.

This keto bowl features a variety of fresh low-carb veggies, satisfying protein and healthy fats that I usually have on hand, and ties it all together with a delicious horseradish mayo.

Ingredients (makes 2 servings)

Power bowl:

- ✓ 1 large salmon fillet, smoked or cooked, flaked (200 g/ 7.1 oz)
- ✓ 1/2 large avocado, sliced (100 g/ 3.5 oz)
- ✓ 2 hard-boiled eggs, halved
- ✓ 2 tbsp raw red onion or Pickled Red Onion (15 g/ 0.5 oz)
- ✓ small bunch of asparagus (100 g/ 3.5 oz)
- ✓ 2 tbsp pumpkin seeds/pepitas (16 g/ 0.6 oz)
- ✓ 1 head of lettuce or salad greens of choice (200 g/ 7.1 oz)

Horseradish mayo:

- ✓ 2 tbsp paleo mayonnaise (30 g/ 1.1 oz) - you can make your own mayo
- ✓ 1 tbsp extra virgin olive oil (15 ml)
- ✓ 1 tbsp apple cider vinegar (15 ml)
- ✓ 1 tsp prepared horseradish
- ✓ 1/2 tbsp capers, chopped
- ✓ 1 tbsp flatleaf parsley, chopped
- ✓ salt and pepper, to taste

Instructions

1. Wash the greens and place in a salad spinner to remove excess water.
2. Add the asparagus to a microwaveable container with a splash of water (about a teaspoon or two) and cook on high for 3 to 6 minutes (depending on the thickness) until vibrant green but still crunchy. Alternatively, boil on the stovetop in a sauce pan filled with water for 4 to 7 minutes.
3. To make the mayo, combine all ingredients and mix well.
4. Layer the salad greens across two bowls. Add half the salmon, avocado, two egg halves, 1 tablespoon of onion, and half of the asparagus to each bowl

on top of the salad greens. Sprinkle with the pepitas. Serve drizzled over the salad.

5. Serve immediately or store in the fridge for up to a day.

8. Low-Carb Caprese Chicken Bowls

These keto Caprese Chicken Bowls are a delicious and □uick lunch option that travels perfectly and packs a protein and healthy fat punch. This recipe is single serving but feel free to increase the amounts as it's super scalable.

It's ultra high in potassium and magnesium and will provide a good amount of protein and healthy fats to keep you satisfied for longer, especially if you are one of those who only eat twice a day.

If you can't find baby mozzarella balls feel free to use fresh sliced mozzarella or even shredded mozzarella in a pinch. If you're making this with plans to travel with it, be sure to store the dressing separately so that the greens don't get soggy. You can toss the avocado with a bit of lemon juice to keep it from browning.

Ingredients (makes 1 serving)

Marinated chicken:

- ✓ 1 small skinless and boneless chicken breast (113 g/ 4 oz)
- ✓ 1 tbsp extra virgin olive oil (15 ml)
- ✓ 1 tsp balsamic vinegar
- ✓ 1 tsp Italian seasoning
- ✓ pinch of salt

Salad:

- ✓ 2 cups fresh spinach or any greens of choice (60 g/ 2.1 oz)
- ✓ 1/4 loose cup basil leaves (8-10 leaves)
- ✓ 6 baby mozzarella balls or fresh mozzarella, sliced (57 g/ 2 oz)
- ✓ 1/2 avocado, thinly sliced (100 g/ 3.5 oz)
- ✓ 1/3 cup cherry tomatoes, halved (50 g/ 1.8 oz)

Dressing:

- ✓ 1 tbsp extra virgin olive oil (15 ml)
- ✓ 1 tsp balsamic vinegar
- ✓ sea salt and pepper, to taste

Instructions

- Place the chicken breast in a sealable container with the olive oil, vinegar, Italian seasoning, and salt. Transfer to the refrigerator to marinate anywhere from 10 minutes to overnight.

- Heat a pan over medium high heat. Transfer the chicken along with the marinade to the skillet and sear 4-5 minutes per side until the chicken is cooked through. Transfer to a cutting board and slice.

- In a small jar, whisk together the dressing ingredients. Set aside until ready to serve.

- Assemble the salads by placing the veggies and mozzarella in a bowl.

- Top with chicken and dressing. Serve immediately.If you're packing the salad to go, store the dressing separately.

9. Keto Fat Head Tricolore Pizza

Fat head dough fan? OMG guys you have to try this low-carb Fat Head chicken tricolore pizza. Cheesy, grain-free and gluten-free keto pizza dough loaded with homemade marinara sauce, succulent chicken, pesto and stringy mozzarella. The perfect Friday night feast.

This keto recipe yields one large pizza. Serve half if you're the one meal a day (OMAD) style keto eater who practices intermittent fasting, or a quarter (2 slices) as a regular meal.

Ingredients (makes 4 servings)

Fat head pizza base:

- ✓ 1 1/2 cups shredded low-moisture mozzarella (170 g/ 6 oz)
- ✓ 2 tbsp cream cheese (30 g/ 1.1 oz)
- ✓ 1 large egg
- ✓ 1/2 tsp sea salt
- ✓ 3/4 cup + 1 tbsp almond flour (80 g/ 2.8 oz)

Pizza topping:

- ✓ 2 small chicken breasts (300 g/ 10.6 oz)
- ✓ 1/4 tsp sea salt
- ✓ pinch of black pepper
- ✓ 1 tsp ghee, duck fat or olive oil

- ✓ 1/4 cup sugar-free marinara sauce (60 ml/ 2 fl oz) - You can make your own marinara sauce in just 5 minutes!
- ✓ 2 balls of mozzarella, sliced (250 g/ 8.8 oz)
- ✓ 2 tbsp pesto (30 g/ 1.1 oz) - you can make your own pesto!
- ✓ 5 pieces sun-dried tomatoes, chopped (15 g/ 0.5 oz)
- ✓ 1/2 cup fresh rocket (5 g/ 0.2 oz)

Instructions

- Preheat the oven to 200 °C/ 400 °F (fan assisted), or 220 °C/ 425 °F (conventional). Place the grated mozzarella cheese into a bowl and add the cream cheese. Microwave on high for 1 minute.
- Mix with a spatula and microwave on high for another 30 seconds and mix. Add the egg and stir. Add salt, almond flour and mix until well combined.
- Place the dough on a heatproof baking mat and use your hands to flatten until about 1/2 - 1 cm (1/4 - 1/2 inch) thick. Alternatively, you can use a piece of parchment paper on top and roll the dough out. If the dough is sticky, use a bit of olive

oil for greasing to dampen your hands when flattening the dough.

- Gently prick the dough with a fork and bake in the oven for 10 minutes until golden.
- Meanwhile, prepare the topping. Season the chicken with a little olive oil, salt and pepper. Grease a griddle pan (or a regular pan) to prevent sticking. Preheat on a medium heat and char-grill the chicken for 4 - 5 minutes each side until cooked through. Remove from the heat and allow to rest before slicing.
- Remove the fathead pizza base from the oven and spread the sugar-free marinara sauce on top. Add slices of mozzarella and chicken breast.
- Place back in the oven for 5 minutes. Remove from the oven and top with fresh sun-dried tomatoes, pesto and rocket.
- Enjoy warm! To store, let it cool down and place in the fridge for up to 3 days.

10. Low-Carb & Keto California Omelet

This keto recipe yields one very large omelet or two small omelets. Feel free to make this quick and serve by cutting in half or if you're the one meal a day (OMAD) style keto eater who practices intermittent fasting, this makes a great large meal! Serve it up with extra hot sauce on the side for a fiery kick!

How to Cook Bacon in a Skillet?

Place the slices in a hot skillet. Add about 1/2 cup (120 ml) water and cook on medium until the water evaporates and the bacon is crisped up, for 10-15 minutes. As the fat renders, the bacon will cook and crisp up in it. Use a slotted spoon to transfer the crisped up bacon to a plate, leaving the rendered fat in the skillet.

If you're using leaner bacon slices, you can lightly grease the skillet with ghee, lard or duck fat and then cook for 2-3 minutes per side until crisp. You can then store your bacon in the fridge for up to four days or freeze for up to three months.

How to Cook Bacon in the Oven?

To cook bacon in the oven, preheat the oven to 190 °C/ 375 °F (fan assisted), or 210 °C/ 410 °F (conventional). Line a baking tray with baking paper. Lay the bacon strips out flat on the baking paper, leaving space so they don't overlap. Place the tray in the oven and cook for about 10-15 minutes until golden brown. The time depends on the thickness of the bacon slices. When done, remove from the oven and set aside to cool down.

Ingredients (makes 2 servings)

- ✓ 6 large eggs, whisked
- ✓ 1/4 tsp lemon juice
- ✓ 1/4 tsp hot sauce (you can make your own Sriracha Sauce)
- ✓ 1/4 tsp sea salt
- ✓ 3 tbsp butter, ghee or duck fat (43 g/ 1.5 oz)
- ✓ 10-12 pieces cooked shrimp, peeled and deveined (115 g/ 4 oz)
- ✓ 2 tbsp minced parsley or cilantro
- ✓ 1/4 cup minced red bell pepper (37 g/ 1.3 oz)
- ✓ 1 medium green onion, sliced (15 g/ 0.5 oz)
- ✓ 1 large avocado, sliced (200 g/ 7.1 oz)

✓ 2 slices cooked bacon (32 g/ 1.1 oz)

Instructions

- In a small bowl whisk the eggs, lemon juice, hot sauce, and salt together. You can make one large omelet and eat half per serving, or make 2 regular omelets.

- Heat the butter in a large nonstick pan over medium-low heat. Once melted pour in the whisked eggs. Cook lifting the edges with a spatula and tilting the pan to allow uncooked egg to run under the omelet until set but still moist on top. If you're making 2 smaller omelets, cook them in batches.

- Arrange the shrimp, parsley, bell pepper, green onion, avocado and bacon across the top of the omelet. Gently fold in half and cook another 2-3 minutes until cooked through.

- Serve immediately.

11. Low-Carb Shrimp Cobb Salad Jars

These easy low-carb Shrimp Cobb Salad Jars are a great packable lunch idea for keto on-the-go! You can prepare these ahead of time up to 2 days in advance. We've chosen to go with a delicious cilantro dressing here but blue cheese or even ranch are equally delicious. If you're not a fan of cilantro, fresh parsley will be just as delicious!

To make these low-carb and keto salad jars super easy, buy pre-cooked shrimp and even pre-boiled eggs if you wish. Otherwise add about 20 minutes to the cook time here. For tips on how to cook the perfect hard boiled eggs and how to make crispy bacon, check out the tips below!

How to Hard-Boil Eggs

To boil the eggs, place them in a pot and fill with water covering them by an inch. Bring to a boil over high heat. Once the water starts boiling, turn off the heat and cover with a lid. Remove from the burner and keep the eggs covered in the pot for 13 minutes (10 minutes for medium sized eggs, 15 minutes for extra large eggs). When done, transfer to a bowl filled with ice water and let them sit for 5 minutes.

To peel, remove from the ice water and crack each egg several times on the kitchen surface. Gently peel off the shells. Fresh eggs don't peel well. It's better if you use eggs that you bought 7-10 days before cooking.

Ingredients (makes 2 servings)

Cobb salad:

- ✓ 8-10 large cooked shrimp/prawns (170 g/ 6 oz)
- ✓ 2 hard-boiled eggs, quartered (100 g/ 3.5 oz)
- ✓ 4 slices cooked bacon, chopped (64 g/ 2.3 oz)
- ✓ 1/2 cup cherry tomatoes, halved (75 g/ 2.6 oz)
- ✓ 1/2 small red onion, sliced (30 g/ 1.1 oz)
- ✓ 1/2 cup diced cucumber (65 g/ 2.3 oz)
- ✓ 1 head Romaine lettuce (200 g/ 7.1 oz)
- ✓ 1 large avocado, diced (200 g/ 7.1 oz)

Cilantro dressing:

- ✓ 1/4 cup extra virgin olive oil (60 ml/ 2 fl oz)
- ✓ 2 tbsp lime juice (30 ml)
- ✓ 1/4 cup chopped cilantro or parsley
- ✓ 1 clove garlic, minced
- ✓ 1/2 tsp ground cumin
- ✓ 1/2 tsp onion powder
- ✓ 1/4 tsp sea salt

Instructions

1. Chop the vegetables. Prepare the dressing by mixing all of the ingredients. If you prefer your dressing super smooth, use a blender and process until smooth.

2. Cook the eggs and crisp up the bacon. To see how you can do that, check the intro.

3. Assemble the jars in this order from bottom to top: dressing, avocado, lettuce, cucumber, red onion, tomato, shrimp, bacon and egg. Season with salt and pepper on top. We used 1-□uart/L, wide-mouth jars because they work best as they are easy to eat from.

4. Store in the refrigerator until ready to eat, no longer than for up to 2 days. Before eating simply give the jar a shake to distribute the dressing. If you prefer to, empty the salad on a plate — as you flip it, the dressing will spread evenly.

12. Keto Buffalo Chicken Chopped Salad

This recipe makes three regular servings or two large servings. A large serving (half of this recipe) is ideal for those who practice intermittent fasting and need a nutritious meal to break their fasting window.

Ingredients (makes 3 servings)

Buffalo chicken:

- ✓ 285 g cooked diced chicken (10 oz)
- ✓ 3 tbsp butter, melted (43 g/ 1.5 oz)
- ✓ 1/4 cup Frank's RedHot sauce or Sriracha chili sauce (60 ml/ 2 fl oz) - you can make your own chili sauce

Salad:

- ✓ 1 large romaine lettuce, chopped (285 g/ 10 oz)
- ✓ 4 slices crisped up bacon, crumbled (64 g/ 2.3 oz)
- ✓ 1 small carrot, diced (60 g/ 2.1 oz)
- ✓ 1/4 cup banana peppers or green bell peppers (30 g/ 1.1 oz)
- ✓ 4 green onions, thinly sliced (60 g/ 2.1 oz)
- ✓ 1/2 cup halved cherry tomatoes (75 g/ 2.6 oz)
- ✓ 1/4 cup crumbled blue cheese (34 g/ 1.2 oz)
- ✓ 1 large avocado, diced (200 g/ 7.1 oz)

Dressing:

- ✓ 6 tbsp ranch dressing (90 ml/ 3.2 fl oz) - you can make your own Keto Ranch Dressing
- ✓ 2 tbsp crumbled blue cheese (20 g/ 0.7 oz)
- ✓ 1 tbsp buffalo sauce or Sriracha chili sauce (15 ml)

Instructions

1. In a medium bowl toss the chicken with the melted butter and buffalo sauce.
2. In a small jar mix together the dressing ingredients.
3. Divide the salad fillings between three salad bowls, top with chicken and drizzle with dressing.
4. Serve immediately or store in the fridge for up to 2 days.

13. Low-Carb Steak Taco Bowl

It's packed with flavor using simple fresh ingredients: cilantro lime cauliflower rice, juicy steak, avocado, sour cream, homemade tomato salsa, crunchy jalapeños, and radishes. Yum! This recipe can easily be scaled up to make multiple servings as well.

Tip: This easy taco bowl is a great option for those who practice intermittent fasting as just one serving will provide enough protein, fat and electrolytes to keep you full and nourished for longer.

Ingredients (makes 1 serving)

Steak Bowl:

- ✓ 1 small filet steak or any of your favorite steaks (150 g/ 5.3 oz)
- ✓ 1 tbsp butter or ghee (15 ml)
- ✓ salt and pepper, to taste
- ✓ 1 cup cauliflower rice, cooked (120 g/ 4.2 oz)
- ✓ 2 tbsp minced cilantro
- ✓ 1 tsp lime juice

Toppings:

- ✓ 1/2 medium avocado, sliced (75 g/ 2.7 oz)
- ✓ 1/4 cup Simple Tomato Salsa or our Radish Salsa or Summer Vegetable Salsa (50 g/ 1.8 oz)
- ✓ 1 tbsp sour cream (12 g/ 0.4 oz)
- ✓ 1/2 jalapeño pepper, sliced (7 g/ 0.3 oz)

✓ 2 radishes, thinly sliced (15 g/ 0.5 oz)

Optional: more cilantro and lime wedges for garnish

Instructions

1. Heat the butter over medium-high heat in a small skillet. Season the filet with salt and pepper. Sear the filet for 4 to 8 minutes per side, depending on how you want the steak cooked.
2. Transfer to a cutting board and allow to rest while you assemble the rest of the bowls.
3. In a bowl, mix the cooked cauliflower rice with cilantro and lime juice.
4. Top with other toppings. Thinly slice the steak and place on top of the cauliflower rice.
5. Serve immediately or store in the fridge for up to a day.

14. Low-Carb Cheese & Bacon Stuffed Meat Pies

These keto meat pies are satisfying enough to be served as a main dish with a side of dressed greens or on its own. It's a great option for those who practice intermittent fasting as it will provide enough fats and protein to break your fast. This recipe makes 6 regular pies (made in an oversized muffin pan) or 10-12 smaller pies (made in a regular sized muffin pan).

Ingredients (makes 6 meat pies)

Filling:

- ✓ 500 g ground beef (1.1 lb)
- ✓ 4 large slices bacon, chopped (120 g/ 4.2 oz)
- ✓ 1 small brown onion, chopped (g/ oz)
- ✓ 1 tbsp coconut aminos (15 ml)
- ✓ 2 tbsp tomato sauce/passata (30 ml)
- ✓ 1 cup beef stock or bone broth (240 ml/ 8 fl oz)
- ✓ 1/2 tsp xanthan gum

Pie crust:

- ✓ 2 1/4 cups shredded mozzarella cheese (250 g/ 8.8 oz)
- ✓ 1 cup + 2 tbsp shredded edam cheese (125 g/ 4.4 oz)
- ✓ 1/3 cup + 1 tbsp full-fat cream cheese (100 g/ 3.5 oz)
- ✓ 1 1/2 cups almond flour (150 g/ 5.3 oz)
- ✓ 2 large eggs
- ✓ 1 tsp onion powder

✓ 6 small chunks of sharp cheddar (66 g/ 2.3 oz)

Instructions

1. Cut the bacon into small strips and dice the onion.

2. Add to a skillet, along with the ground beef. Cook until just browned.

3. Add coconut aminos, passata, beef stock and xanthan gum and stir well to combine. Bring to the boil then reduce the heat and simmer for 30 minutes.

4. Remove from the heat and let cool. Once mixture is cool, heat oven to 200 °C/ 400 °F (fan assisted), or 220 °C/ 425 °F (conventional).

5. Prepare the pie crust. Place the cheeses and cream cheese into a large bowl and microwave for 1 minute. Remove and stir, then return for another 30 seconds. Repeat this once more. Add the almond meal, onion powder and eggs and mix well until you have a soft dough.

6. Divide into four parts and sit one portion aside. Cut each of the remaining three portions in half and then flatten them out into large circles (you will have a total of six circles).

7. Spray a six-hole oversized muffin pan and press the dough into each cup, making sure to leave overhang at the top as the dough will shrink while cooking. Bake for 10 minutes.

8. Remove and spoon some filling in to each cup. Press a chunk of cheddar into the centre.

9. Then top with the remaining filling.

10. Divide the reserved dough into six and flatten out into lids. Lay the lid on top of the pies and gently press around the edges to seal. Cut a couple of steam vents in top of each pie.

11. Return to the oven for 10-15 minutes until golden brown on top.

12. Eat warm, with sugar-free ketchup if you want to feel very Australian. If you can't find sugar-free, you can make your own keto ketchup in just a few minutes! Store in the refrigerator for up to 5 days.

15. Low-Carb Butter Braised Cabbage with Crispy Ham

I heard butter and I heard cabbage and my mind went, hmmmmm... Here is the result, soft, velvety cabbage in a rich buttery sauce.

This high-fat dish is ideal as a side with lean meat cuts such as pork tenderloin, beef sirloin, chicken breasts or white fish. If you practice intermittent fasting and only eat one or two high energy meals per day, feel free to serve it with fatty meat cuts such as pork belly, beef ribeye or fatty fish such as salmon.

Ingredients (makes 4 servings)

- ✓ 1/2 head white or green cabbage (600 g/ 1.3 lb)
- ✓ 2 sticks unsalted butter (225 g/ 8 oz)
- ✓ sea salt, to taste
- ✓ black pepper, to taste
- ✓ 6 slices prosciutto di Parma (90 g/ 3.2 oz)

Instructions

1. Slice cabbage and place it in a dutch oven or large saucepan.
2. Chop butter into chunks and sit on top of cabbage.
3. Put lid on pot and cook on low for about 2 hours, stirring every 15-20 minutes to prevent burning. Do not put water in.
4. Heat oven to 180 °C/ 355 °F (fan assisted), or 200 °C/ 400 °F (conventional). Place prosciutto on a

rack over an oven tray and cook for 10-15 minutes until crispy.

5. Cool, then crumble roughly into a container.

6. Once cabbage is finished, serve with a healthy grind of black pepper and crumbled prosciutto on top.

7. Store in a container in the refrigerator for up to 4 days.

16. Salmon BLT Keto Sandwich

This keto Salmon BLT is an awesome low-carb and grain-free sandwich! There's □uite a few variations you could do as well:

- Mix chipotles in adobo into the mayo
- Add chile powder and lime juice to the mayo
- Add fresh or roasted garlic to the mayo
- Add sliced avocado to the sandwich
- Add a slice of cheese such as cheddar, provolone or manchego

I could go on and on with a million different ideas, leave yours in the comments below!

We used the all-time favorite Keto Buns recipe for the bread here and they are perfect! I love keeping a batch of the on hand during the week for easy sandwiches. This low-carb bread recipe is ideal for meal prep and healthy lunchboxes.

With less than 6 grams of net carbs, over 40 grams of protein and 60 grams of fat, this meal is ideal for those who practice intermittent fasting and need a nutritious meal to break their fasting window.

Ingredients (makes 1 serving)

- ✓ 1 Ultimate Keto Bun - see other suggestions below
- ✓ 1 small salmon fillet (115 g/ 4 oz)
- ✓ 1 tbsp avocado oil, olive oil or ghee (15 ml)
- ✓ 2 slices bacon (60 g/ 2.1 oz)
- ✓ 2 leaves lettuce (10 g/ 0.4 oz)
- ✓ 1 slice tomato (27 g/ 1 oz)
- ✓ 1 slice red onion (8 g/ 0.3 oz)
- ✓ 1 tbsp mayonnaise (15 g/ 0.5 oz) - you can make your own mayo

Note: Instead of keto buns, you can make a regular Keto Bread Loaf and slice to make a sandwich (flax-free and nut-free option included), or Nut-Free Keto Buns if you can't eat nuts.

Instructions

1. Preheat grill pan or skillet to high heat. Season the salmon with salt and pepper. Add the oil to the skillet then crisp up the bacon.
2. Sear the salmon skin side down for 5 minutes until it easily releases from the pan. Flip and cook 2 more minutes. Remove and set aside.
3. To assemble, slice the bun in half and layer in the lettuce, salmon, onion, tomato, bacon, and mayonnaise.
4. Serve immediately.
5. The sandwich is best eaten fresh but can be stored in a lunchbox in the fridge for up to a day. The buns can be stored ay room temperature for up to 3 days, or frozen in a freezer bag for up to 3 months.

17. Spicy Beef Keto Hot Pockets

Ingredients (makes 2 servings)

Filling:

- ✓ 1/2 small brown onion (35 g/ 1.2 oz)

- ✓ 2 garlic cloves (6 g/ 0.4 oz)
- ✓ 1 tsp ghee or butter
- ✓ 300 g ground beef (10.6 oz)
- ✓ 1 - 2 small chile peppers, chopped (10 g/ 0.4 oz)
- ✓ 1 tsp coconut aminos
- ✓ 1 tsp Sriracha sauce (you can make your own Sriracha)
- ✓ 1/4 tsp sea salt, or to taste
- ✓ 1/4 tsp black pepper, or to taste
- ✓ 1 cup fresh spinach (30 g/ 1.1 oz)

Dough:

- ✓ 3/4 cup shredded low-moisture mozzarella (85 g/ 3 oz)
- ✓ 1/3 cup almond flour (33 g/ 1.2 oz)

Instructions

1. Preheat the oven to 200 °C/ 400 °F (conventional), or 180 °C/ 355 °F (fan assisted). Chop the onion and garlic. Heat the ghee in a non stick or cast iron pan on a medium heat.
2. Add the onion and fry for 2 minutes until soft. Add the garlic for a further 30 seconds. Add the beef and cook for approximately 5 more minutes until

cooked through, breaking the mince up with a spatular until fine.

3. Add the chilli, coconut aminos, sriracha and season to taste. Stir through the spinach, cooking for 1 - 2 minutes until wilted. Turn off the heat and place to one side.

4. Melt the mozzarella in a microwave for about 60 seconds until the mozzarella melts. Add the almond flour and mix to combine to form a dough.

5. Roll between two sheets of greaseproof paper or one sheet and a silicone mat.

6. Place the chilli beef mixture in the centre and fold to seal the dough.

7. Careful prick or slice a few air holes in the top.

8. Place on a greaseproof lined baking tray and bake in the oven for 15 - 20 minutes until golden.

9. Best served fresh - enjoy!

10. The pockets can be frozen for 2 months and then placed in the oven to reheat.

18. Creamy Pesto Tuna Salad

Despite the extra effort in preparing the creamy tuna topping, this low-carb salad still comes together in under ten minutes making it a ☐uick and delicious meal for those warmer months.

This keto salad is ideal for lunch boxes and those who practice intermittent fasting. It's high in potassium, magnesium, protein and healthy fats. Just one serving will keep you full until dinner!

Ingredients (makes 1 serving)

Creamy tuna:

- ✓ 1 small tin tuna in oil, drained (95 g/ 3.4 oz)
- ✓ 1 1/2 tbsp paleo mayonnaise (23 g/ 0.8 oz) - you can make your own mayo
- ✓ 1 heaped tbsp full-fat Greek yoghurt, coconut yogurt or more mayo (30 g/ 1.1 oz)
- ✓ 1 tbsp pesto (15 g/ 0.5 oz) - you can make your own pesto
- ✓ 2 tsp fresh lemon juice
- ✓ 1/8 tsp sea salt, or to taste

Dressing:

- ✓ 1 tbsp extra virgin olive oil (15 ml)
- ✓ 1/2 tbsp apple cider vinegar or lemon juice

- ✓ 1/8 tsp sea salt
- ✓ 1/8 tsp black pepper

Salad:

- ✓ 4 leaves iceberg lettuce, torn (60 g/ 2.1 oz)
- ✓ 1 small tomato, sliced (60 g/ 2.1 oz)
- ✓ 1/2 small cucumber, sliced diagonally (80 g/ 2.8 oz)
- ✓ 1/4 avocado, thinly sliced (50 g/ 1.8 oz)

Instructions

1. Make the creamy tuna by mixing all the ingredients in a small bowl, and mashing together with a fork until combined. Add salt to taste.
2. To make dressing, add ingredients to a small jar and shake to combine.
3. Layer the lettuce, cucumber and tomato in a shallow bowl.
4. Top with the tuna mix and the avocado. Drizzle over the dressing.
5. Serve immediately, or store in the fridge for a day. The creamy tuna can be made in advance and stored in a sealed jar in the fridge for up to 4 days.

19.Salmon with Asparagus & Quick Blender Hollandaise

An easy but impressive dish, this low-carb salmon with ⬚uick blender Hollandaise sauce and asparagus is a fabulous dinner that's packed with healthy fats. The creamy hollandaise sauce is 100% foolproof and goes perfectly with the fatty salmon and the crisp asparagus. I choose to use a blender for making the hollandaise and it turns out perfect every time.

The key is to make sure that your butter is super hot and bubbling so that it cooks the egg yolks and turns them into a thick creamy sauce and not runny, using a blender whips a bit of air into the sauce making it extra silky which I love as well.

Ingredients (makes 2 servings)

Salmon & Asparagus:

- ✓ 1 tbsp avocado oil, ghee or extra virgin olive oil (15 ml)
- ✓ 2 small wild salmon fillets (250 g/ 8.8 oz)
- ✓ small bunch asparagus (250 g/ 8.8 oz)

Quick Blender Hollandaise:

- ✓ 2 large egg yolks
- ✓ 6 tbsp unsalted butter or ghee, melted (85 g/ 3 oz)
- ✓ 1 tbsp fresh lemon juice (15 ml)
- ✓ salt and pepper, to taste
- ✓ pinch of cayenne pepper, garlic powder, onion powder or paprika
- ✓ dash of water if too thick

Instructions

1. Heat the oil over medium high heat in a cast iron skillet. Season salmon with salt and pepper and place skin side down in the skillet. Sear 4-5 minutes until the salmon easily released from the bottom of the pan.
2. Flip and continue to sear another 4-5 minutes until it releases again.
3. Flip and place the asparagus in the skillet, cook about 3-4 minutes tossing a few times so each stalk gets a sear on the skillet. Set aside while you make the hollandaise.
4. To make the hollandaise sauce, heat the butter over medium heat until melted and bubbling. Take off the heat.

5. Place the egg yolks in a blender with the lemon juice and cayenne. Blend for 30 seconds until yolks are broken down. With the blender running stream in the bubbling butter in a slow steady stream. The sauce should thicken. If it's too thick, add a dash of water and blend again.

6. Season with salt, pepper and cayenne pepper. Pour over the salmon and asparagus.

7. Serve immediately or store in the fridge for up to a day. Hollandaise is best served fresh.

20. Easy Italian Melt Omelet

There is nothing that I love more than a quick, tasty and filling lunch. Or breakfast.

This low-carb omelette (or omelet for my American friends) is so easy to put together but is full of all of the delicious flavours of Italy. Creamy fresh mozzarella meets salty prosciutto, and they get together with their best friends, tomato and basil, and party together in your mouth.

Ingredients (makes 1 serving)

- ✓ 1 tbsp + 1 tsp extra virgin olive oil (35 ml)
- ✓ 6-8 cherry tomatoes (60 g/ 2.1 oz)

- ✓ 1 tbsp freshly chopped basil
- ✓ 2 slices prosciutto di Parma (20 g/ 0.7 oz)
- ✓ few slices fresh mozzarella (50 g/ 1.8 oz)
- ✓ 3 large eggs
- ✓ salt and pepper, to taste

Instructions

1. Pour 1 tablespoon of the olive oil into an omelette pan and place over medium heat.
2. While heating, quarter the tomatoes, shred the basil and chop the prosciutto and mozzarella into small pieces.
3. Break the eggs into a bowl, season to taste, and whisk until frothy, then pour into the heated pan. Leave to cook for a minute, then run a spatula gently around the underside.
4. Cook until the top and centre look almost set, then scatter the mozzarella, prosciutto, tomatoes and basil over one half of the omelette.
5. Fold the omelette over the fillings, turn the heat off and leave to sit for a minute. Drizzle with the remaining 1 teaspoon of olive oil.
6. Slide the omelette on to a plate and eat while hot. I prefer to eat my omelette when it is fresh

cooked, but you could store it in a covered container in the fridge for up to three days and reheat it prior to eating.

CHAPTER SIX

AUTOPHAGY

Autophagy is a self-digesting mechanism responsible for removal of damaged organelles, malformed proteins during biosynthesis, and nonfunctional long-lived proteins by lysosome. Autophagy has been divided into three general types depending on the mechanism by which intracellular materials are delivered into lysosome for degradation that is, microautophagy, chaperonemediated autophagy (CMA), and macroautophagy. In microautophagy cytoplasm material is sequestered through direct invagination to the lysosomal membrane.

Whereas in CMA proteins flagged with pentapeptide motif (KFERQ) were selectively degraded through direct translocation into lysosome. Macroautophagy involves the formation of subcellular double-membranebound structures called autophagosomes that contain degradable contents of cytoplasm materials and deliver them into lysosomes for breakdown by lysosomal enzymes. The molecular mechanism of autophagy involves several conserved Atg (autophagy-related) proteins. Systems produce modified complexes as autophagy regulators. Autophagy is activated in response to diverse stress and physiological conditions. For example, food deprivation, hyperthermia, and hypoxia are mediated by factors like insulin/IGF-1, m-TOR signaling, FOXO transcription factors, and chaperones.

The perturbance in autophagy may lead to several types of cancers, myopathies, and neuromuscular disorders. Several autophagy inducers and inhibitors like 3-methyladenine (3-MA), bafilomycin A1, LY294002 (LY), and Velcade have been used to treat disease is an intense field of study.

What Is Autophagy?

Before delving into the aspects of autophagy, There is a wellknown answer to the question: What is an autophagy? In the current science, autophagy is a self-digesting mechanism responsible for removal of long-lived proteins, damaged organelles, and malformed proteins during biosynthesis by lysosome. The evidence demonstrates that autophagic process is meant for regulating diverse cellular functions including growth, differentiation, response to nutrient deficit and oxidative stress, cell death, and macromolecule and organelle turnover.

Autophagy Mechanism

Autophagy involves the formation of a double-membrane vesicle, which encapsulates cytoplasm, malformed proteins, long-lived proteins, and organelles and then fuses with lysosomes for degradation. The formation of the doublemembrane vesicle is a complex process involving 16 autophagy-related proteins (Atg proteins). Apart from this, two ubiquitin-like conjugation systems are involved in autophagy. These systems produce modified complexes of autophagy regulators: Atg8-PE and Atg5-Atg12-Atg16, and that may determine the formation and size of the autophagosome. The nucleation, expansion, uncoating, and completion of the autophagosome formation then occur, leading it to fuse with lysosomes.

The molecular mechanism of autophagy involves several conserved Atg (autophagy-related) proteins, most of which were first identified in yeast. Initiation of autophagosome formation requires two complexes. (1) A complex that contains the class III PI3 K Vps34,

Atg6/Beclin1, Atg14, and Vps15/p150.73. (2) The other complex includes a serine/threonine kinase Atg1. The kinase activity of Atg1 requires the function of two other autophagy proteins, that is, Atg13 or Atg8 and Atg17. In mammals, which do not contain Atg13, Atg1 was found to associate with the Atg8 orthologues, LC3 (microtubule-associated protein light chain 3), GATE-16 (Golgi-associated ATPase enhancer of 16 KDa), and GABARAP (G-amino butyric acid type A receptor-associated protein).

The elongation involves two ubiquitin-like conjugation pathways, the Atg8/MAP-LC3/GABARAP/GATE-16 and Atg12 systems. The soluble Atg8 protein undergoes a carboxyl-terminal cleavage by the cysteine protease Atg4 to expose a reactive glycine residue to mediate autophagosome formation. Atg4 is activated by the Atg7 (E1- like) and Atg3 (E2-like) enzymes. The function of Atg3 requires a protein complex which involves Atg5, Atg12, and Atg16. The phosphatidyl ethanolamine is then covalently bound to activated Atg8 (Atg8-PE in yeast and lipidated LC3-II in mammals). It remains bound to the autophagosome membrane until some of it was cleaved by Atg4 to be recycled. If uncleaved by Atg4 it gets degraded within the autolysosome, as Atg8 remains covalently bonded to the membrane and may therefore be used as a marker for autophagy. As soon as autophagosome formation is completed, the Atg16-Atg5-Atg12 complex dissociates from its bordering membrane, and components take part in a recycling process mediated by Atg2, Atg9, and Atg18. Now the completed autophagosome is ready for fusion with the endosome or the lysosome.

Autophagy Regulation

Autophagy is activated in response to diverse stress and physiological conditions. For example, food deprivation, hyperthermia, and hypoxia, which are known as major environmental modulators of ageing, are also conditions that induce autophagy [8–10]. At molecular level, an autophagy pathway displays remarkable interrelations with factors influencing ageing.

Insulin/IGF-1 Regulates Autophagy

The nutrient-responsive IGF-1/Insulin signaling pathway promotes reproductive growth, morphogenesis, and survival. In C. elegans, insulin/IGF-

1 signaling pathway prevents dauer development. In mutants, dauer development is independent of growth conditions like reduced insulin/IGF1 receptor activity. The mutant animals were reported to show high level of autophagy in the cells associated with morphogenesis. The disruption in autophagy gene function inhibits morphogenesis and survival. Certain autophagy genes have been reported to influence on cell growth, the effects being mediated by insulin/IGF-1 or TGF β signaling.

For example, nematodes are unable to grow in giant body size phenotype when autophagy gene activity was disrupted and with aberrant insulin/IGF1 or TGF β receptor activity. This implies that autophagy genes are controlling the cell size converged by the growth modulator signaling pathways. In mammals, the relationship between autophagy and insulin/IGF-1 signaling appears to be more intimate.

m-TOR Regulates Autophagy

Nutrient deprivation or treatment with rapamycin induces autophagy. In yeast, Atg13 is hyperphosphorylated by TORC1 (the rapamycin-sensitive TOR kinase complex 1) and has lower affinity for Atg1. Apart from this, TORC1 controls activation of several effectors that regulate transcription or translation of certain proteins by phosphorylation, some of which are re□uired for autophagy. TOR regulates induction of autophagy in cooperation with two other nutrient sensing pathways, that is, protein kinase A and SCh9. In mammals, mTOR appears to regulate autophagy in similar way to the yeast. Further, AMPK acting at upstream of TOR promotes autophagy in human cell lines and flies. Thus, mTOR along with insulin/IGF1 signaling controls autophagy at several levels. Normal cell growth re□uires a well balance between protein/organelle synthesis and degradation (turnover). Increased growth rate implies accumulation of aberrant cytosolic components.

Irreversibly modified (e.g., oxidised, crosslinked) proteins, malformed proteins, and defective mitochondria act as cellular toxins, which interfere with normal cellular function. These cellular toxins accumulate progressively as the age is advanced, providing a gradually reduced ability of the organisms, normal functions and to survive.

The evidence shows that mammalian target of rapamycin (mTOR) acts as a negative regulator, and the extent of autophagy is regulated by proteins upstream of mTOR signaling, including PTEN, PDK1, Akt, and TSC1/2. For example, PTEN and TSC1/2 positively regulate autophagy, whereas Akt inhibits it. Downstream targets of mTOR, including elongation factor-2 kinase and S6kinase, have been shown to regulate autophagy.

DRAM and Regulate Autophagy

The fact is that p53 suppressor is mutated in approximately 50% of human cancers and induces autophagy. It has been reported that P53 functions as critical mediator for damage-induced apoptosis and has been shown to induce autophagy in DRAM- (Damage-regulated autophagy modulator-) dependent manner to execute a full cell death in human cancer cell lines. DRAM is a lysosomal integral membrane protein, and a direct target of p53-induces macroautophagy and helps in accumulation of autophagosomes. The p53 mediated apoptosis involves several chromatin-remodeling factors (e.g., e2f1 as it involves in transcriptional repression of cell proliferation as part of component with retinoblastoma complex). Autophagy genes may also be controlled by the factors involved in chromatin remodeling as p53 functions at upstream of autophagy pathway to cause cell death. Recent data show that e2f1 binds to Atg1, atg8, and DRAM regulatory regions in human.

Autophagy is a lysosome-mediated degradative process of eukaryotic cells to digest their own constituents during development or starvation. The autophagy has been divided into three general types depending on the mechanism by which intracellular materials are delivered into the lysosome for degradative process:

(1) microautophagy,

(2) chaperone-mediated autophagy (CMA), and

(3) macroautophagy.

In microautophagy, cytoplasmic material is sequestered through direct invagination to the lysosomal membrane. In chaperone-mediated autophagy (CMA), proteins bearing a particular pentapeptide motif (KFERQ) are selectively degraded through direct translocation into the lysosome. This is absent in plants.

Macroautophagy involves the formation of subcellular double-membrane-bound structures called autophagosomes, contains degradable contents to se□uester cytoplasmic materials, and delivers them into lysosomes for breakdown by lysosomal enzymes.

The products of degradation can be reused for cell functioning. The process of macroautophagy (hereafter referred to as autophagy) starts with the initiation of the formation of the isolation membrane (phagophore), a process called nucleation. The growth of the phagophore (elongation or expansion) terminates in the completion of the autophagosome. Then the fusion of the autophagosome with lysosome forms an autolysosome within which the enclosed material is degraded.

Chaperone-mediated autophagy (CMA) is differentiated from other types of autophagy by two properties, that is, its selectivity towards a particular pool of cytosolic proteins and the mechanism of delivery of the substrate proteins to lysosomes. It is estimated that about 30% of soluble cytosolic proteins labeled with CMA target motif pentapeptide KFERQ. Only proteins bearing this particular targeting motif in their amino acid se□uence are selectively recognized by the heat shock cognate protein of 70 kDa (hsc70), the chaperone that mediates their delivery to lysosomes.

Some of the following are identified as substrate proteins that include glycolytic enzymes (glyceraldehyde-3-phosphate dehydrogenase, aldolase, and phosphoglyceromutase), 20S proteasome, transcription factors and inhibitors of transcription factors (c-fos, the inhibitor of NFκB [IκB]), α2- microglobulin, calcium-binding proteins, and proteins associated to vesicular trafficking (αsynuclein).

After the CMA targeting motif is recognized by hsc70, the substrate/chaperone complex is targeted to the surface of the lysosomes where it binds to the lysosome-associated membrane protein type 2A (LAMP-2A), a receptor for CMA. Once bound, the substrate unfolds and crosses the lysosomal membrane assisted by a lysosomal form of hsc70 (lys-hsc70) present in the lumen. CMA substrates access the lysosomal lumen directly across the lysosomal membrane. Transport is saturable which requires a source of energy (ATP) and is temperature dependent (binding occurs at temperatures as low as 10∘C, but transport isonly detected at temperatures above 25∘C).

The selectivity to degrade associated through CMA seems beneficial under specific conditions in which discrimination is re□uired for different types of proteins. During prolonged starvation, the CMA provides the amino acids re□uired for protein synthesis but also favors degradation of unnecessary proteins against that of proteins essential for cell survival. Similarly, during mild oxidative stress or after exposure to protein-modifying toxic compounds, this allows the selective removal of the proteins damaged or altered under these conditions.

Autophagy and Cancer

The cell death alteration in cancer is one of the hallmarks, and these cells are under the pressure of survival. The unsuccess in apoptosis causes these cells to transform and leads to genetic damage and carcinogenesis. There are so much information about mutational and expressional alterations of apoptosis genes, such as Fas and caspases in human cancers. However, data on autophagy genes is more limited than apoptosis. In cancers, ATG2, ATG5, ATG9, ATG12, and UVRAG genes have been reported to be mutated with microsatellite instability. The Atg6 (Beclin1) gene is deleted in some cancers, and rarely point mutation is found in human cancers.

The UVRAG mutated binds with Beclin-1 in gastric and colorectal cancers with microsatellite instability. The antiapoptosis genes are likely to be potential oncogenes, while procell death genes are likely to be potential tumor suppressor genes. There is controversy about the role of autophagy in cancer. Some data favor the idea that autophagy suppresses tumorigenesis, whereas other data suggest that autophagy enhances tumorigenesis and protects tumor cells from cell death.

When primary epithelial cells become immortal, a cell death pathway that involves both autophagy and apoptosis is selectively inactivated. In model systems of mammary acini formation, both apoptosis and autophagy are involved in the removal of epithelial cells to form luminal structures. This suggests that autophagy prevents early steps in epithelial tumor development. Taken together, these data imply that autophagy can both stimulate and prevent cancer depending on the context. To further test this idea, it is much more interesting to study mice with defects in other Atg genes to see if they also have a cancer predisposition phenotype similar to the Beclin-1+/− mice.

ATG5 is a protein involved in the early stage of autophagosome formation. Binding of ATG5 with ATG12 contributes to autophagosome formation, which sequesters cytoplasmic materials before lysosomal delivery. Apoptotic stimuli cleave ATG5 which is subsequently translocated to mitochondria and triggers caspase activation. Expression of ATG5 sensitizes tumor cells to chemotherapy, but silencing of ATG5 results in a resistance to the chemotherapy.

The roles of autophagy in cancer are a topic of intense debate. As mentioned above, autophagy allows a cell to respond to changing environmental conditions, such as nutrient deprivation. On starvation, autophagy is greatly increased, allowing the cell to degrade proteins and organelles and thus obtain a source of macromolecular precursors, such as amino acids, fatty acids, and nucleotides, which would not be available otherwise. Thus, autophagy serves as protective role allowing cells to survive during nutrient deprivation.

How autophagy works

Yes, you can actually train your body to eat itself — and, believe it or not, you want it to. It's a natural process called autophagy (the word literally means "self-eating").

It's one way your body cleans house. In this process, your cells create membranes that hunt down scraps of dead, diseased, or worn-out cells; gobble them up; strip 'em for parts; and use the resulting molecules for energy or to make new cell parts Trusted Source

"Think of it as our body's innate recycling program,"

The benefits of autophagy

There's some evidence to suggest that autophagy ("ah-TAH-fah-gee") plays a role in controlling inflammation and boosting immunity, among other benefits. In one 2012 study on mice, researchers found that autophagy protected against:

- cancer
- neurodegenerative disorders
- infections
- inflammatory diseases

- aging
- insulin resistance

Another study from that year showed how a lack of autophagy can be harmful. Researchers found that removing the autophagy gene in mice caused weight gain, lethargy, higher cholesterol, and impaired brain function. Trusted Source

"Autophagy makes us more efficient machines to get rid of faulty parts, stop cancerous growths, and stop metabolic dysfunction like obesity and diabetes,"

How to kick-start autophagy

"So how do I eat myself?" is a question you probably have never asked, but we're about to tell you how. Autophagy is a response to stress, so you're going to want to put your body through some hardship to drum up a little extra self-cannibalism. As is often the case, short-term discomfort can bring long-term benefits.

"It's our ancestral and evolutionary response to dealing with feast and famine in times of stress," "Since a lot of these things would kill us, like starvation and exercise, it only makes sense that after millions of years we adapted those mechanisms to make them positive."

Here are the three main ways to boost autophagy in your body.

1. Lower your carb intake

There's a great way to activate autophagy without forgoing your favorite rib eye — though you'll probably need to quit candy.

It's called ketosis. The idea is to reduce carbohydrates to such low levels that the body has no choice but to use fat as a fuel source. This is the magic behind the wildly popular ketogenic diet.

Keto diets are high in fat and low in carbs (steak, bacon, and peanut butter shakes are a bonus for the keto crowd). Between 60 and 70 percent of your overall calories come from fat. Protein makes up 20 to 30 percent of calories, while only 5 percent comes from carbs.

Being in ketosis can help people lose body fat while retaining muscle. There's some evidence that it also may help the body fight cancerous tumors, lower the risk of diabetes, and protect against brain disorders, particularly epilepsy. In fact, in a 2018 study, rats fed a keto diet had less brain damage during seizures. "Ketosis is like an autophagy hack,". "You get a lot of the same metabolic changes and benefits of fasting without actually fasting."

If staying in ketosis sounds too hard, take heart. A 2012 study noted similar benefits in people who followed a diet in which no more than 30 percent of their overall calories came from carbs.

Note: Anyone with health issues, especially kidney or liver problems, should talk to a doctor before beginning a keto diet.

2. Try intermittent fasting

Skipping meals is another stressful act that the body may not immediately love but ultimately benefits from. Research has shown there are loads of positives to an occasional fast. One research review found that intermittent fasting and autophagy can make cancer treatments more effective while protecting normal cells and reducing side effects.

In another mouse study, intermittent fasting was shown to improve cognitive function, brain structure, and neuroplasticity, which is fancy-speak for the brain's ability to reorganize and rebuild itself.

That said, it wasn't totally clear if autophagy was the cause. Plus, the study was done on mice. You may have heard about a certain Twitter account that has a problem with people talking big about mouse studies. In the meantime, give fasting a shot. While Champ fasts for 18 hours per day a couple of times per week, he knows that can be a tough routine for most of us.

Different variations of intermittent fasting seem to show pretty awesome health benefits. A review of the research concluded that it may have an array of positive effects, ranging from a healthier body weight and lower risk of diseases to an increased lifespan.

Keep in mind that fasting is generally not recommended for children, for some people with diabetes or other issues with blood sugar, or for pregnant women.

3. Exercise regularly

In case the sweating, grunting, and post-workout pain didn't tip you off, here's the deal: Exercise puts stress on your body.

Working out actually damages your muscles, causing microscopic tears that your body then rushes to heal. This makes your muscles stronger and more resistant to any further "damage" you might cause them.

Regular exercise is the most popular way people unintentionally help their bodies cleanse themselves. (So there's actually something to that fresh, renewed feeling you get after working out.)

A 2012 study looked at autophagosomes, structures that form around pieces of cells the body has decided to recycle. After engineering mice to have glowing green autophagosomes (as one does), scientists found something interesting.

The rate at which the mice were healthily demolishing their own cells drastically increased after they ran for 30 minutes on a treadmill. The rate continued to increase until the little guys had been running for 80 minutes.

So, what about humans?

It's hard to figure out the amount of exercise required to switch on the autophagy boost.

"[These] are hard questions to answer at the moment," says Daniel Klionsky, PhD, a cellular biologist at the University of Michigan who specializes in autophagy.

"Clearly exercise has many benefits, aside from the possible role of autophagy."

Is there an easier way?

Not yet. But there's a lot money to be made if researchers can distill the benefits of autophagy into a pill, so you can be sure they're trying.

"Of course people are looking for ways to induce autophagy through chemicals, because it would be easier than dieting," Klionsky says, but he warns that we're a long way off.

In 2018, for instance, the FDA approved stiripentol, which can imitate the effects of a ketogenic diet. It's used for the treatment of seizures associated with Dravet syndrome, a rare form of epilepsy.

Still, don't get your hopes up. "There are so many metabolic changes that take place during ketosis that mimicking all of them with a pill might not be possible," Champ says. "The bodily stress that comes with entering ketosis might be necessary for the benefits."

Just remember: You don't have to stay in ketosis, fast, or exercise intensely all day, every day to experience these benefits. Even a few hours here and there can help.

CHAPTER SEVEN

SCIENTIFIC STUDIES ON FASTING

Just over a year ago, Alex Allen moved across the country to San Francisco. He'd landed a job as a software engineer, achieving his dream of working in a city at the center of the tech industry. The 24-year-old loved the area's open culture and mild, consistent weather. He wanted to make the most of his adopted city.

But socializing inevitably posed a problem. Sometimes, dinner with new friends meant he sipped water as he watched them chow down.

In the last couple of years, he'd started a fasting diet — 16 hours of fasting and then eating within an eight-hour window each day. It had been a wake-up call for his body. In his late teens and early 20s, he lifted weights regularly, but he also packed on a lot of fat. He was over 200 pounds, and he was tired of it.

So he tried a 16-hour fast, a popular method called 16:8. He experimented with another popular regimen, 20:4, eating within a four-hour window of a 24-hour day. Like a bodybuilder switching to heavier barbells, Allen eventually mixed in daylong fasts to his routine. His weight dropped to 166 pounds within four months.

He stuck to his diet in San Francisco but realized he'd have to just get through that part of sitting down to a meal with people. "It was a bit odd at first," says Allen. "But I don't mind doing it anymore. It starts a lot of conversations."

Fasting began as a way for him to lose flab. It soon became a way of life. "Nowadays, I do it for the other health benefits and just because it makes me feel great," says Allen. Those benefits are more energy, inner calm and mental clarity. "I can't imagine fasting not being part of my routine for the rest of my life."

Allen is part of a growing trend that started several years ago, when fasting caught the public's attention as a weight-loss strategy. Advocates say the practice is easier to stick to than other diet plans. But that alone doesn't account for its staying power. Fasting also has its share of clinical studies to back it up.

Research shows it's an effective weight-loss strategy and also has potential to improve health for people of normal weight. Regular practice may delay the onset of age-related diseases, such as cancer, Type 2 diabetes and neurodegenerative diseases, such as Alzheimer's. It also appears to enhance learning and memory, and can increase life span.

In addition, fasting is being explored as a supplemental treatment for brain injury, various cancers and metabolic syndrome. Most of these results are preliminary, and many of them are conclusions from animal studies.

Still, Valter Longo, a cell biologist and fasting researcher at the University of Southern California, says fasting is the body's built-in fixer. It holds the power to heal. "But now, because we eat all the time, that inner repair has been eliminated," he says. "We are not benefiting anymore from this ability."

Fasting is not the first dietary approach to excite researchers. Before fasting, there was caloric restriction, or CR. The methods have much in common. Overall, they both drastically reduce energy intake and bring about similar health benefits. They're like siblings in a way, especially since fasting studies emerged from work on CR. And now, many former CR researchers are exploring fasting, often setting the two against each other in the lab.

Although CR never caught on with the public like fasting has, it remains an important dietary experiment for scientists studying the biology of aging. To better understand today's fascination with fasting, we first need the skinny on CR.

120 or Bust

Scientists have studied CR for 100 years. In that time, they have realized that lab animals whose daily energy intake was restricted by 20 to 40 percent lived longer and had a lower chance of chronic illness and disease. It was a baffling revelation: Eating less than the body apparently needs is a healthy strategy.

Up through the 1980s, researchers carried out the majority of CR experiments only on yeast, flies, mice and rats. An important question remained: Would CR work in humans?

That opportunity came by chance in 1991, when eight scientists entered Biosphere 2, an enclosed artificial ecological system near Tucson, Arizona. Their mission was to live for two years on food grown within the domed habitat to glean information for future biosphere space colonies.

Physician Roy Walford was one of the scientists. He also happened to be a CR devotee and had recently written a book on living to the age of 120 by following the regimen. Soon after entering, the team realized the food they raised in the dome wouldn't be enough to sustain them. So Walford implemented an impromptu CR experiment. The four men and four women reduced their approximate calorie intake by up to 30 percent. It was essentially the first human study of CR and its effects.

In a paper published in 2002 on the pseudo-experiment, Walford and colleagues reported that the Biosphere staff had been in excellent health. Nearly all of them lowered their blood pressure, blood sugar, cholesterol and other health measures. Still, their skeletal appearance was shocking. "They were malnourished, and they didn't look healthy," says Eric Ravussin, a metabolic researcher at the Pennington Biomedical Research Center in Baton Rouge, Louisiana.

Biosphere 2 helped lay the groundwork for an unprecedented study. In 2008, Ravussin and collaborators put together the first rigorous clinical human trial of CR, called Calerie.

The trial, which aimed to investigate how food deprivation affects the aging process, involved 218 normal and slightly overweight men and women between the ages of 21 and 51. Of the group, 143 of them were tasked with following CR, eating 25 percent fewer calories than usual — a decrease deemed feasible based on animal studies. They were to keep this regimen for two years with help from a behavioral intervention team and dietitians to make sure they were getting basic nutrition.

Most people in the CR group completed the trial, but their average drop in calories was just 12 percent. It didn't matter, though. Blood pressure, cholesterol, glucose, insulin and other biomarkers fell, possibly lowering their risk for heart disease, cancer and diabetes.

After the trial, another research group fed the Calerie biomarker data into age-estimation algorithms; they wanted to see whether CR might have had an effect on longevity. The conclusion was striking: During the study period, the people following CR had aged more slowly than those in the control group.

This mirrored some of what researchers were finding in non-human primates. Rhesus monkeys share 93 percent of their genetic makeup with humans and usually live to about 26 in captivity. In one study on 76 rhesus monkeys that's been running since 1989 at the Wisconsin National Primate Research Center, monkeys on a 30 percent calorie cut lived, on average, two to three years longer than control monkeys. Another ongoing study, started in 1987 by the National Institute on Aging on 121 rhesus monkeys, hasn't detected the same boost to longevity. But CR has worked remarkably well for the 10 males that started the diet later in life. At least four have lived past age 40, including one to 43 — a record for the species.

As Old as Life Itself

Despite the data from studies, scientists still aren't completely sure how and why CR works. It might be an adaptation that developed billions of years ago in microorganisms trying to survive when food was scarce. Studies on E. coli show that when switched from a nutrient-rich broth to zero nutrients, the bacteria live four times longer.

It appears that restricting calories activates genes that direct cells to preserve resources. Rather than grow and divide, cells in famine mode are, in effect, stalled. In this state, they are mostly resistant to disease and stress and enter into autophagy, a process of cleaning out dead or toxic cell matter and repairing and recycling damaged components.

On top of that, in mammals, production of a hormone that's key to cellular growth, called IGF-1, drops, according to several papers. The hormone helps youngsters grow tall and strong, but in adults, it increases cancer risk and accelerates aging when not suppressed.

Jeffrey Peipert wasn't necessarily after any potential anti-aging benefits when he enrolled in the Calerie trial. And he wasn't purely aiming to advance the research on cellular aging. He mostly wanted to lose weight.

Peipert was 48, stood at 5 feet, 5 inches, and weighed 174 pounds. During the trial, he cut his daily food intake from 3,300 to 2,475 calories, and his weight dropped to 147 pounds. His health biomarkers, especially his blood pressure, were excellent. "It was a remarkable drop in blood pressure. That taught me that, for our health, if we were just a little thinner, we'd be better off," says Peipert, a gynecologist and researcher at the Indiana University School of Medicine.

The big takeaway from Calerie, Longo says, is that the biomarkers of health are controllable through weight loss. "So if your doctor is telling you that you need drugs to control these things, that's not true," he says.

Not All Magic

Although CR might be metabolic magic, it's no magic bullet. Some mice bred to carry certain genes for lab research don't benefit from it, and it actually shortens life in other genetically modified mice. The deprivation can weaken the immune system of very young and very old animals, making them susceptible to disease. And although cutting calories by 25 percent has been standard, it's not clear if that's best for animals and humans.

As with mice, people react differently to food deprivation. In recent years, scientists have learned that genetics, diet composition (amount of carbs, protein and fats), regular exercise and other factors play a role in CR's effectiveness.

Peipert's experience in the Calerie trial points to these issues. Despite his banner biomarkers, he had trouble sleeping, a reduced libido, low energy and was hungry most of the time. "I used to love to garden," says Peipert, now 57. But during the trial, "I was wheeling a wheelbarrow around full of dirt, and I felt weak. I wasn't myself."

These types of side effects weren't more common in CR dieters overall, but several people had to pull out of the study because of safety concerns. Noted side effects of CR are chronic loss of bone density and lean body mass, and excessive weight loss. Some CR dieters have body mass indexes in the teens, which suggest malnutrition and frailty, Longo says.

CR can lead to psychological issues, too. These were minimal in the Calerie trial, but Ravussin says that's likely because people were screened for predispositions: food fantasies, irritability and social isolation, he says. Some of the Biosphere 2 scientists said they became prickly and obsessed about food during their 21-month deprivation.

Kelly Vitousek, a psychologist at the University of Hawaii who has written review papers on CR, says these problems make sense from an evolutionary perspective; food is one of our top priorities. "Don't waste your time on other stuff," she says. "Think food, not about socializing, not about sex. Be preoccupied with food. Obtain it."

During the Biosphere 2 experience and the Calerie trial, some researchers hoped CR would become a viable regimen. But the enthusiasm has significantly cooled. While side effects were an issue, people's inability to stick to a significantly reduced calorie load every day was the hammer blow. At this point, fasting was CR's heir apparent: It seems eating nothing on occasion might be better than eating less all the time.

Fasting Redux

Fasting has deep roots in human culture. It's been a practice within various religions for millennia, and the ancient Greeks marveled at its impact on the body and mind. For centuries, doctors noticed it could reduce epileptic seizures. Paracelsus, a 16th-century German-Swiss physician, called it "the physician within."

But it wasn't until the 1940s that the first experiments began as an outgrowth of CR studies. Researchers started withholding food from lab animals on alternate days, says Michelle Harvie, a research dietitian in Manchester, England. And in 1946, The Journal of Nutrition published the first study on fasting, showing that rats deprived of food every third day lived longer and were less likely to develop tumors than control animals. Later work showed that fasting spurs metabolic changes similar to those of CR.

By the 2000s, some fasting studies were showing better results than CR. In a 2003 experiment, Mark Mattson, a neuroscientist at Johns Hopkins University and the National Institute on Aging, found that mice fed on alternate days were healthier than mice that were calorie-restricted by 40 percent.

In 2012, the idea of fasting was popularized when BBC commentator Michael Mosley aired a popular television documentary about the diet. A best-selling book, The Fast Diet, followed the next year.

As fasting has grown in popularity, scientists and nutritionists have developed different methods of the practice. Some, such as Allen, practice time-restricted feeding, like the 20:4 regimen. Some push the approach to 23:1, cramming all their eating into one hour of a 24-

hour day. Other approaches space out fasting days throughout the week, such as the 5:2 method — two days of fasting over seven days. Some enthusiasts supplement their practice with dayslong fasts.

Although people normally think of fasting as only consuming water, the most popular of these plans does allow for calories on "fast" days — just not enough to impede the practice's healthy physiological effects, says Mattson.

In 2012, Carolyn Corbin, who lives in the Channel Islands, got some firsthand experience with fasting's flexibility. At 5 feet, 2 inches tall and 159 pounds, Corbin was overweight, with a BMI of 29.1. After seeing Mosley's BBC show, she took up the 5:2 regimen, eating 500 calories two days a week and eating normally the rest of the time. She soon switched to water-only fasts two days a week. Since taking up the practice, the 65-year-old has lost 35 pounds and kept it off. "Forget calorie counting, diet food and diet drinks," Corbin says. "Fasting for weight loss works."

And there's more than anecdotal experience like Corbin's that fasting can help people lose weight. In a one-year study, 100 obese adults ages 18 to 64 were assigned to three groups. One group practiced alternate-day fasting, eating 75 percent fewer calories every other day; another group followed CR, with a 25 percent calorie restriction every day; the rest were in a control group. Compared with the control group, the fasters averaged 6 percent weight loss, and those assigned to CR averaged about 5 percent, according to the 2017 paper in JAMA Internal Medicine.

Even with these results, one of the concerns with fasting is that people will binge on non-fast days. But the results of two months-long trials, published in 2018 in the journal Food Science & Nutrition, showed that dieters, specifically those following 5:2, didn't binge. "When you impose a two-day 70 percent calorie restriction, what they do on the natural days is eat about 25 percent less," says Harvie, one of the authors of the study and a co-developer of the 5:2 diet. "And that is why the diet is so effective."

Fast Lane

Popular Water-Only or Low-Calorie (500-600) Fasting Plans:

1. **Time-restricted feeding:**

Eating within a specific window of time in a 24-hour period. The most popular is 18:6, eating only during a six-hour period of a 24-hour day. Other variations are 20:4, 22:2 and 23:1.

2. **Alternate-day fasting:**

Fasting every other day.

3. **Intermittent fasting:**

Fasting one day or several days a week. Most popular is 5:2 — eating normally five days a week, fasting two days a week.

The Ketone Connection

Is fasting better at improving people's health than CR? It's far from clear. However, rodent experiments suggest it might be better at enhancing cognition. For years, researchers have seen mice and rats perform well on cognitive tests when famished. While on alternate-day fasting, rodents improve their endurance, senses, memory and ability to learn.

So what accounts for this heightened mental state? It seems fasting triggers a dramatic switch in the body's metabolism, according to a paper Mattson and colleagues published in February in the experimental biology journal FASEB. In humans, fasting for 12 hours or more drops the levels of glycogen, a form of cellular glucose. Like changing to a backup gas tank, the body switches from glucose to fatty acids, a more efficient fuel. The switch generates the production of ketones, which are energy molecules that are made in the liver. "When the fats are mobilized and used to produce ketones, we think that is a key factor in accruing the health benefits.

One type of ketone flooding the brain is beta-hydroxybutyrate, or BHB. According to a paper published in February in Nature Reviews Neuroscience, BHB stimulates memory, learning and the cellular housekeeping process of autophagy in mice. BHB also triggers neurons, including those in the hippocampus, a memory center in the brain, to release what's called brain-derived neurotrophic factor, or BDNF, a protein that is important for learning, memory and improved mood. CR doesn't generate these levels of ketones because glucose stores are never empty.

Mattson points out that, from an evolutionary perspective, the brain power that fasting generates makes sense. Mammals typically go days without food, often hunting on an empty belly. Semi-starved animals with enhanced smarts and energy would be more likely to obtain food and live another day. "If you are that wolf or lion, now a week with no food, you better be able to focus your mind and concentrate on what you need to do to get food," he says.

Ketones might also help explain several mysteries surrounding brain injuries and disorders. For instance, fasting rodents recover more fully from brain trauma and spinal cord injury, according to several studies.

Feast or Fad?

But fasting comes with its own caveats: a higher risk of binge eating, low blood pressure, irritability and headaches. The latter two tend to go away after a few weeks, as the body adjusts to fewer calories. Still, dayslong fasts can cause fainting spells. Doctors recommend it only under the guidance of a physician.

Ravussin, the CR researcher, isn't convinced fasting offers more benefits than CR, or that ketones are as powerful as Mattson and Longo say. "Ketones are a good thing to curb your appetite, but are they a good thing as far as cellular health?" he asks. "I have not seen convincing data that says yes."

Harvie believes fasting might be here to stay, partly because it's flexible. People can choose a fasting practice and nutrient plan that fits their lifestyle, she says. "We twitter on about which diets are better. But at the end of the day, a diet is only as good as the person who follows it," says Harvie. "For some people, the 5:2 will be perfect, and for others, it will be absolutely awful."

Vitousek, the psychologist, has seen this kind of enthusiasm before — and it was for CR. Caloric restriction never reached fasting's popularity, but it had its share of lay followers in the 2000s, when she got a chance to talk with members of a group practicing it. Initially, they were excited and motivated. Then, like most dieters, the majority began to fall away. Some who had done CR for years simply couldn't do it anymore. "You can pretty much take that to the bank," Vitousek says of dieters' waning enthusiasm. "That's why we have these cyclical waves."

For Peipert, it's been a seesaw journey. He's always struggled with his weight, and obesity runs in his family. A few years after the Calerie trial, he regained all the weight he'd lost, plus 6 pounds. "That kind of drastic calorie reduction for two years is probably not a sustainable or good plan for lifelong weight loss," he says.

When fasting emerged as a diet, Peipert was skeptical. But in March, he started the 5:2 regimen. It was hard at first, he says, but by midsummer, he'd lost 9 pounds. He hopes to lose 10 to 15 more. "It has helped me control my hunger," says Peipert. And with his experience of CR still on his mind, "No side effects."

Fasting Shortcuts

Even though fasting and caloric restriction can offer health benefits, both re□uire eating less — something unappealing to most people. So scientists and nutritionists have experimented with ways to mimic the biochemical and physiological effects brought about by sustained periods of food deprivation.

Keto Diets Ketosis occurs when the body, deprived of food for 12 hours or more, switches its energy source from carbs and glucose to fatty acids. The process generates ketone bodies that may have healthy effects.

Keto diets, composed of low-carb, high-protein and high-fat foods, can also spark this metabolic switch.

Since the 1920s, keto diets have been used in medicine to reduce epileptic seizures. More recently, the diets have supplemented standard treatments for Type 2 diabetes and cancer, with promising results.

Over the last few years, keto diets have gained mainstream popularity. Some celebrities and sports stars embrace them, and people who fast use the regimen to further push their body into ketosis.

But followers beware, says nutrition researcher Michelle Harvie. Dieters going keto tend to lose weight, but the diets are low in fiber and high in saturated fat, which is a risk for cardiovascular disease. "And there is increasing evidence that its effect on the gut microbiome is pretty adverse," says Harvie. "The gut microbiome is a poorly understood but potentially important part of our metabolic health. And if you mess that up, you're in trouble."

Fasting-Mimicking Diet Valter Longo, a cell biologist at the University of Southern California, has developed ProLon, a five-day diet that mimics a five-day fast, but without loss of essential nutrients. It's an all-vegan diet with high unsaturated fat (think almonds, avocados and peanut butter), low sugar and low protein.

In a 2017 study in Science Translational Medicine, 71 participants who completed the fasting-mimicking diet showed health benefits including weight loss, lower blood pressure and a drop in levels of the hormone IGF-1, which primarily stimulates growth but also plays a role in regulating blood glucose levels. And depending on how healthy you are, you may not need to stick to the diet too long. For instance, Longo says a healthy athlete may need to do it only twice a year, while someone who's overweight may need to continue with it until they see the improvements they want.

Pharmacology Medicines that treat chronic medical conditions, like epilepsy and Type 2 diabetes, are being explored to mimic fasting. The major players are rapamycin, metformin, resveratrol and hydroxycitrate. The drugs show promise, but also have downsides.

Rapamycin, for example, tricks cells into thinking they're nutrient-deprived, sparking the cellular rejuvenation seen in fasting, but it also suppresses the immune system. That's helpful in medical scenarios, such as preventing organ rejection after a transplant or to treat autoimmune diseases, but not so great for the average dieter.

CHAPTER EIGHT

INTERMITTENT AND DISEASE

Fasting, or not eating food for an extended period of time, is well-known as a religious diet practice. But some are also beginning to use it for specific health benefits. Over the past several years, many studies have been published showing that intermittent fasting or a fasting-mimicking diet can reduce risk factors for and reverse symptoms of serious health conditions including cancer and some other diseases that will be mentioned below.

1. CANCER

Your body is designed to protect you against starvation. To do this, it stores a reserve of the nutrients needed to survive when you eat. When you're not eating normally, this puts the cells under mild stress, and your body begins to release those stores to fuel itself. Doctors suggestTrusted Source that as long as your body has time to heal itself after this period of stress, you won't experience negative effects.

One of the most immediate results of this type of diet is weight loss, since your body is using more calories than it's taking in. It's important to be careful about fasting for an extended period of time that your body cannot handle. Complete or continuous fasting will trigger "starvation mode," in which your body starts slowing down to prolong your life. This typically begins after three days of continuous fasting. During this fasting period of more than three days, your body will hold on to fuel stores as much as possible, and you won't notice weight loss.

Weight loss is just one benefit of intermittent fasting for a normal healthy (disease-free) adult. Recent animal studies and a few preliminary human trials have shown a decrease in risk for cancer or a decrease in cancer growth rates. These studies indicate this may be due to the following effects from fasting:

- decreased blood glucose production
- stem cells triggered to regenerate the immune system
- balanced nutritional intake
- increased production of tumor-killing cells

In one study of time-restricted feeding during 9–12 hour phases, fasting was shown to reverse the progression of obesity and type 2 diabetes in mice. Obesity is a major risk factor for cancer, which may support fasting to treat cancer.

A second study of mice showed that a bimonthly fasting-mimicking diet reduced the incidence of cancer. Results were similar in a pilot trial by the same scientists with 19 humans; it showed decreased biomarkers and risk factors for cancer.

Research showed that a combination of fasting and chemotherapy slowed the progression of breast cancer and skin cancer. The combined treatment methods caused the body to produce higher levels of common lymphoid progenitor cells (CLPs) and tumor-infiltrating lymphocytes. CLPs are the precursor cells to lymphocytes, which are white blood cells that migrate into a tumor and are known for killing tumors.

2. TYPE-2- DIABETES

In recent years, intermittent fasting has emerged as a novel way of treating patients with type 2 diabetes. There are anecdotal reports of patients who have lost weight, their blood sugar levels have improved significantly, and they no longer need to take their diabetes medications. Their disease appears to be in remission – if not exactly cured.

However, endocrinologists – the doctors who routinely treat diabetes – as well as dietitians, are skeptical. They point to a lack of major studies that prove this approach is effective and safe long term. After all, intermittent fasting reuires a big change in eating habits and it remains to be seen how many people can stick with it.

The first thing you need to know is that there are different ways of doing intermittent fasting – which is basically not eating for certain periods of time. For instance, you could restrict your consumption of food to just eight hours a day – say from 11 a.m. to 7 p.m. – and eat nothing else for the other 16 hours.

Type 2 is the most common form of diabetes accounting for 85 to 90 per cent of cases. It usually develops later in life and it's often associated with being overweight.

A major feature of the disease is a condition known as insulin resistance. Insulin is a hormone that moves glucose (sugar), from the bloodstream into the body's cells where it is used for energy. For a variety of reasons that are not fully understood, the body's tissues don't respond ade□uately to insulin and glucose then becomes elevated in the bloodstream.

Poorly controlled blood-sugar levels can lead to a host of medical complications, increasing the risk of heart attack, stroke, kidney failure, blindness and limb amputation. Diabetes is often treated with medications to make the body more responsive to insulin. Some patients also take additional insulin to top up the amount produced by their own bodies.

3. EPILEPSY

Reducing calorie intake, or fasting, may help decrease the frequency of seizures in people with epilepsy by calming overexcited neurons in the brain, early research suggests. fasting is known to have health benefits, with those who practice it often living longer. But whether those benefits might extend to the nervous system is a question.

Epileptic seizures are caused by excessive electrical activity within networks of neurons in the brain. This electrical activity is created by the flow of charged particles, or ions, entering and leaving the surface of the neurons. Ions enter and leave via ion channels (like highways), and once the current within the neuron reaches a certain level, it fires signals to axon terminals, or synapses. Synapses are essentially narrow gaps between axon terminals, across which signals are transmitted. Signals cross synapses as a chemical, called a neurotransmitter.

Neurotransmitters can be either excitatory or inhibitory, meaning neurons will be either stimulated to fire or silenced. The main excitatory neurotransmitter is glutamate, and if there is too much of it, neurons can become hyperexcitable and seizures result. A seizure may also arise from too little GABA, the major inhibitory neurotransmitter in the brain. So, in order for the brain to function normally, a fine balance between excitation and inhibition must be maintained.

The research team used fruit fly larvae to show how acute fasting lowered synaptic activity at the neuromuscular junction — where neurons meet muscle cells to control their contraction — in a study representing the entire nervous system. Specifically, they looked at what was previously known about TOR proteins, which are able to increase synaptic activity. TOR is known for increasing cell metabolism by blocking the action of another protein, 4E-BP, a metabolic inhibitor.

4. Alzheimer's Disease

The greatest risk factor for Alzheimer's disease and dementia is aging, and research in aging biology suggests that caloric restriction (i.e., reducing caloric intake by 20–40 percent) may mitigate some of these risks. If caloric restriction can slow the body's aging, there is a chance that it could delay age-related diseases such as Alzheimer's. So how can we reap the potential benefits of caloric restriction? It would be difficult for a healthy person to eat 20–40 percent fewer calories each day throughout life. But previous studies have found that intermittent fasting may have a similar effect.

Intermittent fasting, as the name implies, involves reduced calorie intake or full fasting for 16–24 hours, followed by regular eating. Preclinical studies in rodents suggest that long-term intermittent fasting might promote longevity, reduce cognitive deficits, improve cognition, and increase the generation of new brain cells.

While these studies are promising, no human clinical studies have confirmed that intermittent fasting or even standard calorie restriction promotes brain health or prevents dementia. Preliminary observational evidence and a small randomized controlled trial have suggested some protection from diabetes and cardiovascular disease, two age-related diseases often associated with an increased risk of dementia. And other studies are underway on specific types of intermittent fasting. The Fasting Mimicking Diet was developed by Dr. Valter Longo and involves eating a reduced number of calories on five consecutive fasting days each month in the form of a proprietary solution of micronutrients. And the 5:2 fast diet, now in clinical trials, involves reducing caloric intake to only 500–600 calories, two days per week. None of these studies are focused on dementia prevention or brain health.

Experts in aging biology and genetics do caution that intermittent fasting may be unsafe for certain people, including those with a very low BMI or diabetics receiving insulin or insulin-like drugs. And elderly people are at a greater risk for malnutrition, which research shows may exacerbate frailty, itself a risk factor for dementia. Therefore, reducing caloric intake or fasting may not be advisable for the elderly.

5. Cure Parkinson's Disease

Parkinson's is a neurodegenerative disease that primarily affects the brain's neurons. There are many signs of Parkinson's, including tremors or shaking, trouble moving and loss of one's sense of smell. The disease may also contribute to the development of dementia.

Fasting, ketogenic diets and other approaches may help reduce the symptoms of Parkinson's and other brain diseases, in much of the same way that exercise helps.

You've probably heard that fasting can cleanse your body and improve your health. But did you know that it might help people manage the symptoms of neurodegenerative disorders including Alzheimer's and Parkinson's?

Fasting helps turn fat into ketone bodies — encouraging a healthy transformation in the structure of synapses that are critical for learning and memory, as well as overall brain health.

Resarchers suggests two ways to try out a calorie-restricted diet. First, there's the 5:2 diet. On two nonconsecutive days each week you consume a total of 500 calories each day. On the other five days, just stick with a normal diet. This is usually around 2,000 calories for women or 2,500 for men.

The second option is to experiment with a time-restricted diet, where you condense eating into a single eight-hour period every day. This gives your body the remaining 16 hours to begin burning fat and creating ketones. Also recommends beginning slowly. Start with moderate fasting one day per week. Once your body gets used to it, add a second day. Symptoms such as headaches, lightheadedness, and grouchiness are common in the beginning but typically pass.

6. Polycystic Ovary Syndrome (PCOS)

Polycystic ovary syndrome (PCOS) is a common endocrine system disorder among women of reproductive age. In several cases, PCOS women show infertility or subfertility and other metabolic alteration, such as insulin resistance (InsR), dyslipidaemia, hyperinsulinemia and obesity. Despite the aetiology of the syndrome is still far from be elucidated, it could be considered the result of concurrent endocrine modifications, lifestyle factors and genetic background.

In particular, accumulating evidence suggests that InsR and compensatory hyperinsulinemia play a pivotal pathogenic role in the hyperandrogenism of many PCOS phenotypes, which in turn have a clear detrimental effect on chronic anovulation. Different forms of fasting, such as intermittent fasting (IF, including alternate day fasting, or twice weekly fasting, for example) and periodic fasting (PF, lasting several days or longer every 2 or more weeks) are currently being tested in several in vitro and in vivo studies. Changes in the circulating levels of Insulin Growth Factor-1 (IGF-1), Insulin-like Growth Factor-Binding Protein 1 (IGFBP1), glucose and insulin are typical effects of fasting which may play a key role on aging and metabolic homeostasis. Considering the paramount importance of InsR and compensatory hyperinsulinemia, different fasting regimens can reduce IGF-1, IGFBP1, glucose and insulin levels and consequently have beneficial effects on ovarian function, androgen excess and infertility in PCOS women.

For so many of us living with PCOS, we know all too well that it is so tricky to lose weight with PCOS and we seem to put it on so easily. It is so frustrating! And we have been told over and over again that we need to lose weight and "we'll be fine" but nobody actually tells us how to lose weight with PCOS.

7. Multiple Sclerosis

Multiple sclerosis (MS) is a chronic inflammatory disease of the central nervous system (CNS) and both environmental factors and genetic background affect its development. Due to the fact that MS is more prevalent in western countries, scientists have started to hypothesize that dietary habits could play an important role in MS risk. However, solid scientific data regarding the relationship between nutrition and MS pathogenesis is lacking.

The researchers previously showed that fasting can reduce MS-like symptoms in mice by inducing metabolic and physiological modifications, with an associated modulation of endogenous corticosteroids and systemic adipokines. Based on these previous findings, the researchers wanted to better explore the role of calorie restriction in the clinical course and pathology of the experimental autoimmune encephalomyelitis (EAE) model and in a small pilot trial with patients with relapsing-remitting MS.

CHAPTER NINE

MOST COMMON MISTAKES AND HOW TO FIX THEM

Intermittent Fasting can be an excellent tool when it comes to health and maintaining a healthy body weight - but there are some common pitfalls to avoid. Some people come into difficulty with Intermittent Fasting because they approach it in the wrong way, being aware of the right methods when undertaking Intermittent Fasting can be the difference between success and failure.

Here are the top five mistakes that I see people making all the time when they are fasting:

1. Using it as an excuse to eat rubbish

Unfortunately, people think that intermittent fasting is a magic pill that will solve all their problems. Yes, it is an incredibly effective tool to take control of your health but it won't cancel out eating a diet full of processed foods and sugar. When you are intermittent fasting it is even more important to nourish your body with nutrient dense, whole foods.

When you are in the fasted state, your body starts to break down damaged components and then uses them for of energy, this process cleans and heals the body. It also means your body becomes more sensitive to the food you eat, this is great if it's full of nutrients to nourish the body, but not good if you are eating rubbish.

Not only that, if you aren't nourishing yourself with nutrient dense foods, you will feel hungry all the time – your body will crave nutrients.

2. Trying to calorie restrict during the 'eating window'

One of the main issues that some people face when they start IF is that they continue to calorie restrict when they have broken their fast. The whole point of eating in this way is to listen to your body and start eating until you feel full.

Your body is an amazing machine, if you allow it to do its job properly. Your body will release hormones to make you feel full when it knows it's had enough food. If you calorie restrict during your eating window you may well end up under eating which causes lots of unwanted changes in the body, and long term is not good for you.

3. Attempting to do too many things at once – over train, under eat and try fasting

If you have spent a number of years eating badly and not exercising and you would like to try IF, don't bite off more than you can chew (pun intended!) at the start. Ease yourself into fasting and training gradually; don't start training five times per week, fasting every day and restricting calories when you do eat from day one.

The combination can lead to problems. Your body thrives with a little bit of physical stress here and there but too much stress can create chronic issues.

4. Obsessing over timings and 'eating windows'

In my opinion, one of the main benefits of IF is teaching you to become completely in tune with your body and understand what I call 'real hunger' – something that occurs every 16-24 hours, not every four hours.

Your body should dictate when you should eat, not the clock. If you focus on time periods, you end up counting down the hours until you can eat – you never learn to understand your bodies signals.

5. Not drinking enough water

When your body is in the fasted state it starts to break down damaged components and detoxifies the body. It is very important that you flush out those toxins by drinking lots of water. Ideally, you will drink more water than you usually would. I drink roughly four-fiver liters every day, most of that during my fasting period.

Not only that, drinking water, particularly sparkling water can help you to feel full, which is important when you are first getting into IF.

CHAPTER TEN

BENEFIT OF INTERMITTENT FASTING FOR WOMEN OVER 50

As we sal past 50, we tend to keep an eye out for things that will improve our aging experience, from serums and supplements to diets, drugs, and doctrines. The products on the market are truly endless, but as it turns out, one of the best things you can do for your aging body doesn't involve buying--or buying into--anything.

You may have heard of intermittent fasting, which involves manageable, alternating periods of eating and not eating, aka fasting. The research is pretty clear that intermittent fasting is beneficial in many ways, and this may be especially true for older adults.

Here are five benefits of intermittent fasting, along with how to do it:

1. **Intermittent fasting initiates cellular repair processes in your body.**

Cellular damage is par for the course as we age, but fasting has been shown to induce your body's cellular repair processes, improve hormone function, and even improves the function of genes related to disease protection and longevity.

2. **Intermittent fasting promotes weight loss-- especially belly fat.**

Belly fat is an indication of visceral fat, which lies deep inside the abdominal cavity, surrounding your organs and contributing to disease. Losing belly fat is tough, especially as we age, but according to a recent literature review, intermittent fasting can lead to a loss of four to seven percent of your waist circumference.

A recent study found that intermittent fasting can cause overall weight loss of three to eight percent over three to 24 weeks.

3. Intermittent fasting reduces inflammation and oxidative stress.

Inflammation and oxidative stress are major contributors to disease as we age, and they contribute to the visible signs of aging.

Intermittent fasting reduces markers of oxidative stress and inflammation in overweight adults, according to a study by Louisiana State University Medical Center.

4. Intermittent fasting may help prevent Alzheimer's disease.

A large body of research shows that intermittent fasting is good for the brain, promoting the growth of new nerve cells, protecting against brain damage resulting from stroke, and increasing levels of a hormone called brain-derived neurotrophic factor or BDNF.

A recent study found that intermittent fasting also delayed the onset of Alzheimer's or reduced its severity. Other studies show that intermittent fasting may offer protection against Parkinson's, Huntington's, and other neurodegenerative diseases.

5. Intermittent fasting may extend your life.

A range of recent studies have also found that intermittent fasting extended the participant's lifespan. One study found that rats fasting every other day lived 83 percent longer than non-fasting rats. Additionally, the rate of aging was slowed in the fasting rats, and their body weight and growth rates were reduced.

Is Intermittent Fasting Healthy?

Is intermittent fasting safe? Remember that you're only supposed to fast for twelve to sixteen hours and not for days at a time. You've still got plenty of time to enjoy a satisfying and healthy diet. Of course, some older women may need to eat frequently because of metabolic disorders or the instructions on prescriptions. In that case, you should discuss your eating habits with your medical provider before making any changes.

Woman Eating FruitWhile it's not technically fasting, some doctors have reported intermittent fasting benefits by allowing such easy-to-digest food as whole fruit during the fasting window. Modifications like these can still give your digestive and metabolic system a needed rest. For example, "Fit for Life" was a popular weight loss book that suggested eating only fruit after supper and before lunch.

In fact, the authors of this book said that they had patients who only changed their eating habits with this twelve- to sixteen-hour "fruit" fast each day. They did not follow the diet's other rules or count calories, and they still lost weight and got healthier. This strategy might have simply worked because the dieters replaced junk food with whole foods. In any case, people found this dietary change effective and easy to make. Traditionalists won't call this fasting; however, it's important to know that you may have options if you absolutely can't abstain from food for several hours at a time.

Typical Intermittent Fasting Results

Dr. Becky, a chiropractor and over-50 fitness consultant, says it's tough to find any downsides to IF in the medical literature. She explained that during the fasting period, your blood sugar and insulin levels will drop to low levels. Without insulin's hormonal fat-storing signal, your body will rely upon stored fat for energy.

You can also find an overview of women's health-related intermittent fast results published by the National Library of Medicine. Some highlights of this report include studies on the use of fasting as a tool to reduce the risk of cancer, diabetes and other metabolic diseases, and heart disease.

Is Intermittent Fasting the Best Fat-Loss Tool for You?

In any case, IF appears to work mostly because people find it fairly easy to adhere to. They say it helps them naturally limit calories and make better food choices by reducing eating windows. Some studies suggest that IF is better than only cutting calories, carbs, or fat because it appears to promote fat loss while sparing lean muscle mass.

Of course, most people use IF with another weight-loss plan. For instance, you might decide to eat 1,200 calories a day to lose weight. You may find it much easier to spread out 1,200 calories within two meals and two snacks than in three meals and three snacks. If you've struggled with weight loss because your diet either didn't work or was simply too hard to stick to, you might try intermittent fasting for □uicker results.

CONCLUSION

If I had to sum up intermittent fasting in a few rules I would say this

1. Eat sometimes but not all the time
2. When you do eat, pick the most nutritious foods
3. Indulge in your favorite foods every now and then
4. Remember to exercise.
5. "Smile, breathe, and go slowly."

It's simply one of many lifestyle strategies that can improve your health. Eating real food, exercising and taking care of your sleep are still the most important factors to focus on. If you don't like the idea of fasting, then you can safely ignore this article and continue to do what works for you.

At the end of the day, there is no one-size-fits-all solution when it comes to nutrition. The best diet for you is the one you can stick to in the long run. Intermittent fasting is great for some people, not others. The only way to find out which group you belong to is to try it out.

If you feel good when fasting and find it to be a sustainable way of eating, it can be a very powerful tool to lose weight and improve your health.